THE ECONOMICS OF
PUBLIC SCHOOL
FINANCE

A Rand Educational Policy Study

THE ECONOMICS OF PUBLIC SCHOOL FINANCE

Aaron Samuel Gurwitz

BALLINGER PUBLISHING COMPANY
Cambridge, Massachusetts
A Subsidiary of Harper & Row, Publishers, Inc.

International Standard Book Number: 0–88410–859–7

Library of Congress Catalog Card Number: 81–20552

Printed in the United States of America

Library of Congress Cataloging in Publication Data
Gurwitz, Aaron S.
  The economics of public school finance.

  Bibliography: p.
  Includes index.
  1. Education—United States—Finance. 2. Public schools—United States—Finance. I. Title.
LB2825.G86   379.1'21'0973   81–20552
ISBN 0–88410–859–7   AACR2

DEDICATION

To Susan Abramowitz

CONTENTS

LIST OF FIGURES

LIST OF TABLES

PREFACE

As the twentieth century's third major school finance reform movement approaches its tenth anniversary, it is becoming more and more apparent how difficult it really is to design and build a sound fiscal foundation for public education. One reason that the reform process is so difficult is that courts and legislatures are attempting to influence one part of a complex and rapidly changing economy. Courts and legislatures can control only a very small portion of the numerous independent decisions of families, firms, and educators, all of which influence the flow of funds to public schools. These decisions and their interactions are the stock-in-trade of economists.

Economists alone cannot improve the ways schools are financed, but no one trying to improve school finance should try to do so without the counsel of an economist. Unfortunately, economists are not always easy to work with. They tend to assume a lot, not only about the world but about the knowledge of their audience. They often present what appear to be the most arcane results in the most abstruse language. This book is intended to ease the working relationship between economists and laymen interested in school finance.

The first part of this book presents in some detail the aspects of economic theory most likely to be of use in analyzing school finance systems. The second part casts the general problem of reforming school finance in the framework most amenable to economic analysis and presents a summary of the most relevant economic research. Three appendixes report the most recent economic thinking on some technical problems that arise in designing school finance systems.

This study, which originally appeared as a Rand Corporation Note, was prepared with the financial support of the National Institute of Education. In addition to providing support and encouragement, several members of the NIE staff, most notably James Fox, Lauren Weisberg, and David Mandel, provided numerous comments and suggestions which improved earlier drafts. Once the study had been completed, The Rand Corporation provided the additional financial support required to turn the manuscript into a book. Several of my colleagues at Rand devoted much more than the requisite time and effort in helping me improve the original product. Dennis DeTray and Kathleen Lohr gave me highly detailed critical comments on an earlier draft and most of their excellent suggestions were incorporated. Erma Packman's careful editing improved the clarity of the explication severalfold. Typing by Barbara Eubank and Rosalie Fonoroff highlighted the mistakes it was my job to correct. I am almost left feeling that the remaining errors are my only contribution.

Aaron Samuel Gurwitz
Washington, D.C.

INTRODUCTION

The ultimate purpose of this study is to help improve the school finance system of the United States. An individual can do little, however, to change this large and complex institution for the better. The most one can hope for is to establish an intermediate objective that appears both attainable and useful. The intermediate goal of the study, then, is to facilitate communication between economists and other professionals involved in school finance analysis and policymaking.

THE NEED FOR BETTER COMMUNICATION

Economists have been thinking systematically for 200 years about the issues that confront the school finance system today. In *The Wealth of Nations*, the paradigm of modern political economy, Adam Smith devoted considerable attention to issues of taxation and the role of governments, and an entire chapter to the question of the best way to finance education.

Neither Smith nor anyone else has been able to design a "best possible" school finance system. We are all very much in the dark as to how elementary and secondary schools should be financed. Nevertheless, economics has much to offer to the common search for insights. The more economists and professionals of other disciplines work together, the better their common understanding will be.

A common effort requires communication in two directions. Economists, who tend to theorize about ideal worlds, can benefit from the discipline of close association with policymakers and other analysts who demand that the economists pay attention to current policy issues and feasible alternatives. A school finance analyst or policymaker who understands both the value and limitations of economic analysis will be better able to provide economists with the restraints they need. In the other direction, economists can provide useful advice, mostly cautionary, to others involved in school finance issues. Economists have developed a facility for detecting the blind alleys of policymaking and for assessing the unintended consequences of public policies.

School finance analysts and policymakers have not always taken advantage of the contributions that economists could make in this field. Several states have in recent years undertaken major reforms of their school finance systems. These reforms have absorbed a great deal of tax money and legislative energy. In most cases, expenditure disparities have not been significantly reduced, nor has the burden of taxation necessarily been shifted from the poor to the rich (Carroll 1979).

At the same time, a number of economists have been trying to figure out ways in which states could redistribute educational resources and tax burdens. The results of the most recent of these analyses indicate that the well-intentioned legislatures had, indeed, adopted relatively ineffectual approaches. The policies they chose could not have led to the results they desired, although other policies might have. If legislative staff or other analysts involved in the process had been familiar with the relevant economic literature before they acted, better policy might have been made.

If policymakers have better access to economic analysis, they will, it is hoped, make fewer mistakes in policy, and the search for improved school finance systems will be faster and less expensive.

It has been somewhat difficult for economists and other professionals to communicate. The results of much economic analysis are presented in scholarly journals and expressed in mathematical terms and jargon that are not always comprehensible to those not trained in economics. Part of the failure to communicate is the fault of the economists who have not bothered to translate their findings into common language. However, the many results of economic research refer to subtle and difficult concepts. If the economist must explain each finding from its conceptual beginning, both he and his audience are likely to lose patience with the process before the import of the research is conveyed.

The immediate objectives of this study, therefore, are to make it easier for economists and other professionals to work together to improve school finance in the United States. One way to do this is to develop a common vocabulary, describe a set of basic concepts, and explain the more useful technical tools of economic analysis as applied to school finance. In a sense, this is an economic primer. More important, it identifies the things that economic analysis can do well and the things that it cannot do well, so that the reader will be better able to interpret and judge other work reported in the literature on these topics. Economic analysis can provide insights into how institutions work; it cannot solve social problems. The working relationship will be better if policymakers and analysts know what and what not to expect from economists.

THE AUDIENCE AND THE LEVEL OF DIFFICULTY OF THE STUDY

This study is aimed at a specific audience, namely, individuals who spend a significant part of their work time at least thinking about school finance issues. It is written in particular for legislators on education committees, staffs of such committees, school finance activists and lawyers, researchers in both the economic and education fields, graduate students in a variety of disciplines who are studying related issues, and, in general, anyone who frequently is involved or interested in the analysis of school finance.

The study presents material at a fairly high level of sophistication and goes as far as it can using mathematics no higher than intermediate algebra. Because new and difficult concepts are presented briefly, some parts of the text may require considerable concentration. This choice of level of sophistication may be justified on the grounds that although most specific research findings in the economics of school finance are subject to much more facile explanations than are presented here, a more casual approach would not meet the study's objectives.

Each economic analysis of a specific question is based on a common, unified, general theory of behavior. The full import of any research finding does not become clear until it is understood in the context of this general theory. Since the objective of this study is to enhance communication, and not merely explain individual research projects, author and reader together must work through the theory and only then go on to discuss school finance.

THE CONTENTS OF THE STUDY

The study is divided into two main parts. Part One presents the basic theory of economics: the general model of production and exchange. It then isolates the several aspects of this theory that are most relevant to the analysis of school finance. Individual chapters cover the theories of educational expenditures, taxation, and school district governance.

Part Two presents an economic analysis of school finance reform. The reader should not expect every topic discussed in Part One to lead to some specific insight in Part Two. Rather, the first part provides the conceptual context for economic analysis and prepares the reader to understand future research on school finance, as well as the specific analysis presented in Part Two. Chapters in Part Two cover the objectives of school finance reform, the constraints on reform, the responses of social institutions to reform, and the economic literature on relevant topics.

The text concludes with three appendixes on special topics and technical issues, including cost-of-education indexes, the special problems of cities, and the measurement of inequality.

THE ECONOMICS OF
PUBLIC SCHOOL
FINANCE

THE ECONOMIC THEORY OF PUBLIC SCHOOL FINANCE

1 THE ROLE AND METHODS OF ECONOMIC ANALYSIS

Lawyers, policy analysts, educators, sociologists, political scientists, and economists all contribute to current discussions of public school finance in the United States. The economist's role in the development of better finance mechanisms is a natural one because much of the discussion involves such economic variables as wealth, income, taxes, and public expenditures. This chapter discusses the essential contribution that economists can make and describes the methods they use.

FUNDAMENTAL CONCEPTS OF ECONOMIC ANALYSIS

Model Building

Economists build simplified models to help them organize their thinking about human behavior and the economy. They are interested specifically in how scarce goods and services are produced and distributed among individuals and households. A simplified model of the most important relationships under investigation enables them to understand aspects of an otherwise incomprehensibly complex social system. Such a model consists of explicit, highly general assumptions

3

about the behavior of the economic actors—firms, households, governments, and so forth—involved.

Some economic assumptions used in models are patently unrealistic. Such assumptions are made, however, to simplify an initial analysis of a complex phenomenon. Once the simple case is worked out, the simplifying assumption is replaced by a more complex model. This strategy is used at several points in this study. For example, we assume initially that a dollar buys the same amount of educational services in all school districts. We know that this is not true, but we can gain useful insights by assuming at first that it is true and later in the study analyzing the effects of different costs of education among school districts.

Other model assumptions are fundamental and are retained. Economists assume that people are rational and that they try to live as happily as possible by using what they have as efficiently as possible. Although such assumptions may also seem unrealistic, they enable economists to understand and predict economic outcomes. Economists can understand more and predict better if they make these assumptions than if they do not make them.

Once assumptions have been made, the economist analyzes the model. Conclusions based on the assumptions show how economic outcomes—the observed prices and quantities of goods and services and their distribution among households—depend on specific empirical facts. For example, one widely used model of the behavior of local governments indicates that expenditures per pupil in local schools depend on, among many other things, the distribution of income of the community's residents.

Predictive Theory, Econometrics, and Normative Theory

Model building and analysis—or "predictive economic theory"—is one of three major lines of economic inquiry. Predictive theory generates qualitative predictions of the relationships among economic variables. One such qualitative prediction might be that the more unequal the distribution of income in a community, the lower the expenditures per pupil in local schools will be. Theory alone, however, cannot go beyond these qualitative predictions.

To determine the exact quantitative relationship between, say, the inequality of the income distribution and per pupil expenditures, economists must rely on a second line of inquiry, "econometrics." Econometricians develop and apply statistical techniques to test the hypotheses of predictive economic theory. Econometric models— that is, economic models translated into statistical form—add quantitative content to the qualitative predictions generated by theory.

Criteria for evaluating economic outcomes—known as "welfare economics" or "normative economic theory"—constitute the third line of inquiry. Here the objective is to show how such statements as "We should spend more on the education of poor children than of rich children" derive from specific theoretical assumptions, empirical facts, and value judgments. Welfare economists also have developed a number of highly general evaluation criteria based on certain widely, but not universally, accepted value judgments.

The Application of Economic Analysis to Public School Finance

Each of the major lines of economic analysis discussed above can be useful to policymakers and analysts involved in the complex issues of public school finance in the United States.

Anyone attempting to analyze as complex a social institution as public school finance must have some implicit, simplified model of that system in mind. A single human mind could not comprehend all of the facts and possibilities constituting the actual school finance system. To organize one's thinking about such a system, some simplifying assumptions must be made. Usually these assumptions are implicit, but they nonetheless influence the conclusions that are drawn about how the system operates. For example, when one speaks of school districts "responding" to changes in state or federal regulations, one necessarily must be assuming something about how the individual actions of all of the people who constitute the school district are resolved in a single, final response. Different sets of assumptions about the choices of individual actors and the ways in which these might combine will generate different predictions of how the district will respond.

Economists, like other social scientists, are trained not only to make assumptions and build their own models but also to expose and scrutinize the assumptions in other people's models. Economic theorists can be useful in the development of public school finance policy by exposing the fundamental premises of the policy and showing how the assumptions determine the conclusions.

Welfare economists have a particular role to play. In fact, the entire involvement of economists in school finance analysis can be seen as an exercise in applied welfare economics. Any evaluative statement about school finance systems or outcomes depends on behavioral assumptions, assumptions about specific empirical facts and value judgments. Later we shall see, for example, the assumptions and judgments that underlie the statement that the current school finance system is inequitable because identical tax rates raise different per pupil expenditures in different school districts.

Econometricians play a role in predicting the likely range of outcomes of a variety of proposed changes in current school finance practice. Of course, no econometric model generates perfectly accurate predictions, but econometric statistical techniques lead to more precise predictions than do ad hoc approaches.

Finally, economists' skills can be applied to some of the technical problems involved in school finance. The development of cost-of-education indexes or inequality measures may be straightforward applications of one aspect or another of economic theory.

THE BASIC MODEL OF PRODUCTION AND EXCHANGE

An economist confronting a specific problem creates his own model. However, all models developed by economists are based on a general underlying theory of production and exchange. The elements of this theory and their interactions are illustrated in Figure 1–1.

Households, Firms, and Governments

The fundamental model describes the characteristics and behaviors of three groups of actors: households, firms, and governments. All are discussed in this chapter; later chapters treat the role of governments in greater detail.

Figure 1–1.   Model of production and exchange

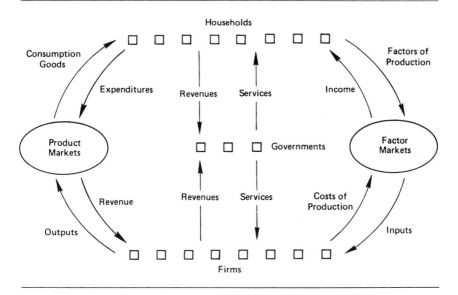

Economists assume that each household or individual owns a given quantity of each "factor of production." A factor of production may be an area of land, a machine, a quantity of raw materials, or an individual's ability to perform labor. The initial distribution of these factors of production among households is assumed to be given, although as the economic system operates through time the distribution of factors of production among the households may change.

Each household or individual is also characterized by a given set of tastes or preferences for certain combinations of "consumer goods." Finally, households are assumed to behave so as to maximize their "utility," that is, their well-being or happiness. They do this by selling or renting out their factors of production and using the income from these sales to purchase consumer goods. Typically, a household sells labor time, receives wage income, and buys consumer goods. Or the household may rent its capital—machines, land, and so on—to producers and use the capital income to buy consumer goods.

Consumer goods are produced by the second set of economic actors, the firms. The firms producing each product are assumed to be characterized by a given production technology, defined as all of the possible ways of producing any given quantity of the product. Firms behave so as to maximize profits. They buy some combination of factors of production to use as inputs and sell some quantity of output. They choose the input combination that minimizes the cost of producing the output and sell just the amount of output to produce the greatest profit.

Three additional sets of basic assumptions complete the model. First, economists assume that substitution is possible in production and consumption: that equal quantities of output can be produced with different combinations of inputs and that equal levels of well-being (utility) can be achieved with different combinations of consumer goods. For example, it may be assumed that 500 bushels of corn can be produced with either one acre of land and one person-year of labor or with one-half acre of land and five person-years of labor, other factors of production held constant. Or, it may be assumed that a household can be equally happy with either a television tape machine or a two-week trip to Europe, other household consumption held constant.

Economists also assume the existence of institutions of exchange, or "markets," where factors of production are exchanged for consumer income and where the outputs of firms are exchanged for revenue. These market institutions are assumed to work in such a way that the quantity of each good brought to the market for sale, the "supply," just equals the quantity that buyers want to buy, the "demand."

The price mechanism insures that the supply will equal the demand. If, at some price per unit, the quantity demanded of a good exceeds the quantity supplied, the price rises. Producers of the good are then induced to produce more of it; consumers, deciding to substitute some other good for the now more expensive one, demand less.

Finally, economists assume that only the relative prices of goods matter to consumers or producers. If all prices were suddenly to double, including the prices of factors of production, it is assumed that the consumption decisions of households and the production decisions of firms would remain unchanged.[1]

1. This assumption allows economists to separate issues related to consumption and production decisions from the highly complex theory of inflation. A great deal of economic analysis deals with the effects of inflation on the behavior of firms and households. Certainly, if inflation affects some prices more than others, people's choices will change. For example, if the price of labor rises more slowly than the prices of consumer goods, the effect is to decrease consumer income. Inflation and policies intended to reduce inflation affect schools, along with all other institutions. School revenues may increase more or less rapidly than the prices of the inputs that schools use, but these effects are subtle and difficult to analyze. This study therefore ignores these effects in presenting a broad picture of how school finance institutions work.

Allocations of Goods

The process of exchange results in the "allocation" of goods among consumers and households. An allocation represents a list for each consumer or firm in an economy of the quantities of each factor of production or consumer good used by that firm or consumer. Figure 1–2 shows the form of a simple allocation. Goods (commodities), the outputs of firms and the factors of production, are listed across the top. Firms and households are listed vertically. This matrix filled in with a set of numbers would represent an allocation of goods and services. The operation of the market system generates both prices for each of the commodities and the allocation of quantities of goods. Either outcome—prices or allocations—may be the object of economic investigation.

Welfare economists have established two basic criteria for evaluating allocations: "efficiency" and "equity." One allocation is said to be better than another if it is more efficient, more equitable, or both. Allocation A is more efficient than allocation B if both are technically feasible and at least one person is subjectively better off under A than under B, while no one is worse off under B.

Figure 1–2.   Allocation of goods

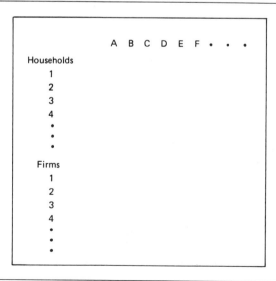

The efficiency of an allocation is an objective criterion; the equity, a subjective one. If one could know how well-off each household was under each of two allocations, everyone would agree on whether one allocation was (objectively) more efficient than the other. People might reasonably disagree, however, about which of two allocations was the fairer, or the more equitable. An individual confronted with alternative allocations would rank them according to his own (subjective) preferences. This ranking would reflect the individual's values.

If these subjective social values display certain general characteristics, welfare theoreticians are able to represent them in a mathematical form, called a "social welfare function." There may be as many different social welfare functions, or value systems, as there are individuals in society. Among all technically feasible allocations (i.e., allocations of goods that can be produced given existing technology and available factors of production), one allocation will be ranked highest by any given individual. This allocation maximizes social welfare. Again, the allocation that maximizes social welfare from the point of view of one individual may differ from that of any other individual.

Analysis of the Model

The analysis of the basic model of production and exchange—the subject of much of the literature on economic theory—indicates that in this system each element of the outcome depends on all other elements of the outcome.

The prices of consumer goods depend on the prices of factors of production in two ways. The incomes of consumers are determined by the payments they receive when they sell their factors of production. Consumer income influences the demand for different commodities and, therefore, helps determine the prices of those commodities. At the same time, since factors of production are purchased by firms and used to produce consumer goods, the prices of the factors determine the cost of production. Cost, in turn, influences the supply and the market price of the good.

Furthermore, when consumer goods are closely related, the price of one influences the prices of the others. Coffee and tea provide a typical example of a close relationship. When the price of coffee rises, many consumers drink tea instead. The increased demand for tea may then be expected to result in higher tea prices. For other goods, the relationship may be extremely tenuous. The price of socks, for example, has little bearing on the price of chewing gum.

PARTIAL EQUILIBRIUM ANALYSIS: SUPPLY AND DEMAND CURVES

The distinction between closely related goods and unrelated goods is reflected in the distinction between partial and general equilibrium models. "Partial equilibrium" models focus on the market for a single good and on how changes in either the supply of or demand for the good influence its own price. Since no single market is perfectly isolated from all other markets, partial equilibrium analysis, which assumes away interrelationships among goods, is always somewhat wrong. However, if a commodity is in fact relatively isolated and if expenditures on that commodity consume a fairly small proportion of the typical family budget, the inaccuracies of partial equilibrium analysis may not matter. Partial equilibrium analysis has the advantage of being easier to do and generating much more clear-cut conclusions than the more complex general equilibrium analysis.

The manipulation of "supply and demand curves" in partial equilibrium analysis is an integral part of economic discourse. Figure 1–3 illustrates a typical supply and demand case. The demand curve slopes downward, reflecting the fact that, typically, when the price of a good goes up, the quantity that consumers will buy decreases. At price P_1, consumers will buy Q_3, but at P_2 they will buy only Q_2. The upward slope of the supply curve illustrates the tendencies of firms to offer more for sale when the price goes up. At P_1, firms will offer only Q_1, but at P_2, they will offer Q_4.

Price does not always determine either the supply of or demand for a given commodity. No matter how high the price goes, the supply of land within three miles of the Chicago Loop is fixed. For other commodities, however, even a small price change will radically alter the quantity supplied or demanded. If a commodity, such as a two-week vacation on one of several identical Caribbean islands, has a perfect substitute, a small increase in the price will cause demand to vanish.

The responsiveness of demand or supply to price is called the "elasticity" of demand or supply. If demand (supply) does not respond to price, the demand (supply) is said to be inelastic. Figure 1–4

Figure 1–3. Typical supply and demand curves

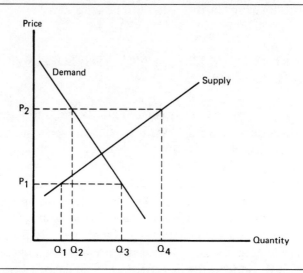

illustrates a price-inelastic demand curve. Demand or supply that responds to price changes is said to be elastic. Figure 1–5, depicting a highly elastic supply curve, indicates that if the price were to rise above P* by even the smallest amount, the supply of the good would

Figure 1–4. Inelastic demand curve

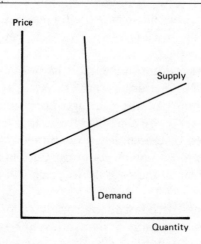

Figure 1–5.   Elastic supply curve

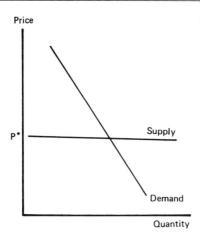

expand by a huge quantity. If the price were to drop slightly below P*, none would be supplied.

Elasticities also have an algebraic representation. The elasticity of demand (or supply) is represented as a percentage change in quantity demanded (supplied) when the price changes by 1 percent. Demand elasticities are usually negative numbers, because when price increases, the quantity purchased goes down. A demand elasticity of −0.2, for example, indicates that the quantity demanded will decrease by 0.2 percent when the price increases by 1 percent. Supply elasticities are usually positive, since the quantity supplied increases when prices increase.

Demand and supply curves are drawn under the assumption that everything in the economy, except the price and quantity of the single good under consideration, remain constant. A change other than in the price or the quantity of the good will induce a shift in the position of either the supply curve or the demand curve or both. Suppose, for example, that the overall income of consumers increases (that is, they now receive a higher price for the factors of production they have to sell), while all other prices in the economy remain the same. For the typical good, this increase will cause a rightward shift in the demand curve. The shift reflects the fact that, at a given price, consumers will now demand a larger quantity of the good than they did when their incomes were lower. Likewise, if the price of important inputs in the

Figure 1–6. Rightward shift in demand curve as result of increased income; leftward shift in supply curve as result of increased production cost

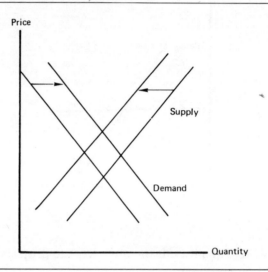

production of the commodity increases, firms will supply a smaller amount of the good at any given price than they did when input prices were lower. This decrease in the quantity supplied at any given price is represented by a leftward shift of the supply curve. These shifts are depicted in Figure 1–6.

Other aspects of supply and demand curves are discussed in greater detail at various points in later chapters.

GENERAL EQUILIBRIUM ANALYSIS

Models of the allocation of goods that are not isolated from other commodities, or that consume a large proportion of the typical family income, cannot safely rely on partial equilibrium analysis. Because they must take into account the interrelationships among all of the closely related commodities, analysis of such markets requires a "general equilibrium" approach.

Consider automobiles. People buy automobiles largely, although not entirely, to provide transportation. How much the number of cars demanded can be expected to change when the price of an average car goes up depends on whether alternative modes of transportation may become available. If alternative transportation is inelastically supplied—that is, if the cost of providing alternative transportation is high—then even large increases in the price of automobiles might induce only small changes in the number demanded. In other words, the elasticity of supply of alternative transportation influences the elasticity of demand for automobiles. An analysis of the market for automobiles must take this relationship into consideration.

The purchase of automobiles consumes a significant proportion of many households' total income. If automobile prices go up and if families are unable to substitute cheaper transportation, they will have to forgo other forms of consumption. The shift in demand patterns will influence other markets, some of them only peripherally related to automobile markets. An analysis of the effects of an increase in automobile prices also must account for these effects on other markets.

When dealing with closely related goods or with goods that consume large portions of the typical family's budget, the economic methodology of choice is general equilibrium analysis. Unfortunately, the economics profession has produced relatively few examples of applied general equilibrium analysis. The problem lies in the complexity of the models. When more than two markets must be taken into account, the number of factors that must be considered so complicates the resulting models as to make it impossible to draw unambiguous or relatively satisfying conclusions. Some "two-sector" general equilibrium models have generated interesting qualitative conclusions. These models treat the relationship between supplies of and demands for two related commodities. We will refer to some of these models in the discussion of the property tax. Researchers recently have had some success in computer simulations of multimarket general equilibrium models. However, general equilibrium analysis of problems in applied economics remains more the ideal than the typical practice. General equilibrium considerations usually take the form of caveats regarding partial equilibrium analysis of specific economic problems.

The basic theory of general equilibrium nevertheless influences the approach of most economists to the identification and analysis of economic problems. Because some knowledge of this theory will enable the noneconomist to better understand the economist's contribution to the discussion of public school finance, we will consider it here in some detail.

General equilibrium theory begins by adding several assumptions to the basic model of production and exchange. At more advanced stages of analysis some of these assumptions are dropped to make the model more realistic. General equilibrium theorists assume, first, that there are markets for everything. For example, they assume that there would be a market for clean air. Second, they assume that consumers' tastes and firms' production technologies satisfy certain technical conditions. They assume further that individual firms and consumers are small and that the total market for any good is large. That is, each firm produces and each consumer buys or sells only a small proportion of the total quantity of each commodity or factor of production traded. This assumption guarantees perfect competition by eliminating individual control over the price of any commodity: No economic actor has any control over the total quantity of a good supplied or demanded at any given price.

Finally, and most important for purposes of school finance analysis, economists assume that there are no "public goods." In the case of private goods, each person's consumption dimishes the total quantity of that good available for other people's consumption. My consumption of a loaf of bread means that there is that much less bread available for others to consume. This is not the case with public goods. Typical examples of public goods are national defense and the Grand Canyon. The protection I receive from our national defense establishment does not reduce the total quantity of protection available to everyone else, nor does my enjoyment of the canyon reduce the amount of canyon left for everyone else to enjoy. In fact, certain aspects of education involve public goods. At this stage of the analysis, economists have assumed away these aspects of the problem.

General equilibrium theorists have proved that, if these assumptions hold, the allocation of goods and services generated by free exchange will be efficient. It would be impossible to rearrange the allocation generated by markets without making at least one consumer worse off. Furthermore, if these assumptions hold, the social welfare evaluation of the resulting allocation depends entirely on the initial distribution of factors of production (wealth) among the households. If, from some individual's subjective point of view, the initial distribution of wealth was "right," then from that individual's point of view the resulting allocation will maximize social welfare. All that would have to be done to generate the best possible allocation would be to redistribute the factors of production initially and then simply to let free exchange operate. The outcome would then be both efficient and equitable.

Of course, the assumptions leading to these conclusions do not, in fact, hold. There are not markets for everything. From an economist's point of view, the pollution problem in the United States reflects the absence of specific markets for a clean environment. The existence of monopolies in some sectors of the economy belies the assumption of perfect competition. Nor are all goods private. Economic theory indicates that when assumptions do not hold, the allocation generated by the free operation of exchange markets may not be efficient and social welfare, from anyone's point of view, may not be maximized.

THE ECONOMIC ACTIVITY OF GOVERNMENTS

Governments play a role in three phases of the economy—allocation, redistribution, and stabilization—that would not function efficiently and equitably without the intervention of a centralized decisionmaker.

The inability of free markets to generate an efficient allocation when there are incomplete markets, monopolies, or public goods calls for government intervention. Governments correct market failures by directly allocating nonmarketed goods—for example, by deciding how much clean air there should be and requiring its provision or by creating artificial incentives that induce firms and households to supply that quantity of clean air. Governments directly produce certain other goods, such as national parks and public education. Governments also are involved in regulating the behavior of monopolies or potential monopolies.

Because decentralized market activities cannot be both efficient and equitable unless the initial distribution of factors of production has been equitable, governments try to insure the equitable distribution of wealth by taxing some people and distributing income or goods to others. The Social Security system and the public housing program both redistribute. Public education is also a redistributive program to the extent that the taxes that poor people pay seldom cover the cost of educating their children.

Finally, governments seek to stabilize the economy. Large, complex economies are subject to severe fluctuations in aggregate economic activity. The federal government attempts to dampen these fluctuations, or at least to minimize the social disruptions that accompany booms and recessions.

To achieve an allocation that is both efficient and equitable, governments first must attempt to find out exactly what consumers want—for example, the right amount of clean air or national defense from each individual's point of view. Since the preferred level of clean air or national defense is likely to differ from individual to individual, governments must find a way to reconcile diverse preferences. In other words, governments must establish rules that will combine and reconcile many different individual social welfare functions. Official social welfare functions—i.e., some aggregation of individual values—inform the government's allocative and redistributive policies. Governments must, in addition, collect tax revenues for allocation (to buy the right amounts of clean air, national defense, and so on) and for redistribution (to support the needy). The choice of the best tax system also involves the process of ascertaining, combining, and reconciling individual preferences.

One branch of economic theory, "public finance," dealing with the taxing and spending behavior of governments, seeks to discover which kinds of government behavior are better or worse than others. The next several chapters apply some of the findings of public finance theory to the issues involved in public school finance.

SUMMARY

Economists build models of the behavior of households, firms, and governments. These three sets of actors exchange factors of production and outputs by means of a system of markets. Market exchanges allocate goods among households.

Economic analysis includes three major activities. Predictive economic theory generates statements about the qualitative relationships among economic variables, such as prices and quantities. Econometrics adds quantitative content to the results of theory by applying statistical techniques to economic models. Normative economic theory develops criteria for evaluating the performance of the economy, comparing alternative allocations according to a social welfare function—a mathematical statement representing an individual's or group's social values.

Analysis focusing on the market for a single commodity—partial equilibrium analysis—is usually represented by sets of supply and demand curves. Information about these two curves can be summarized in a single number called the elasticity. An inelastic demand curve reflects the unresponsiveness of the quantity of some good purchased to the price of the good. An elastic supply, to give another example, indicates the responsiveness of the quantity of a good brought to market for sale to the price of the good.

General equilibrium models represent the relationships among the markets for several commodities. Such models are necessarily so complex as to preclude the use of general equilibrium analysis in most applications. The analysis of general equilibrium theory predicts that, under a set of very unrealistic assumptions, a free market economy will make all consumers as well off as they possibly can be. One of the assumptions behind this conclusion is that there are no public goods.

A public good is such that one individual's consumption of it does not diminish the amount of that good available for others to consume. An example is national defense. If there are public goods, then a free market economy will not generate the best possible economic outcomes, and some government intervention may be called for.

2 THE NORMATIVE THEORY OF EDUCATIONAL EXPENDITURES

This chapter reviews the theory of education as an economic good and two approaches to identifying the optional allocation of education among individuals.

The economic theory of general equilibrium tells us that, given complete markets, perfect competition, and no public goods, free production and exchange generate efficient economic outcomes. The theory holds further that if these outcomes are not the most desirable from a social welfare point of view, it is only because the underlying distribution of factors of production is undesirable.

Economists of education doubt that a completely free educational market, with each household buying just the amount of education it wants and can afford, will generate an efficient and equitable allocation of education. This doubt stems from their evaluation of education as a public good.

EDUCATION AS A PUBLIC GOOD

Economists of education have identified at least three ways in which education generates a public good.

First, the general level of public education benefits each individual in society. Each driver, for example, is likely to be safer when all other drivers are able to read traffic signs. Each resident of a community is likely to be healthier if all other residents understand the basic principles of sanitation. Each citizen is likely to enjoy more responsible government services if all other citizens are able to evaluate the claims and promises of political candidates and vote intelligently.

Second, education is one mechanism through which the shared norms and common experiences that contribute to social cohesion and stability are inculcated. Thus, education may be said to generate the public good of social cohesion and stability.

Third, education may help to redistribute economic outcomes, namely, income and well-being. One way to reduce income inequality is to give some people more education than they would choose, or be able, to purchase in a perfectly free market.[1] By improving the individual's work skills, education enables him to earn a better living and thus also may improve the quality of his life.

Each person consumes, in some sense, the average level of education of the community or nation. Furthermore, the benefit that one individual derives from the general level of education does not diminish the benefit that anyone else derives from generalized literacy, factual knowledge, political acumen, social stability, or equality of economic outcomes. The general level of educational attainment in society is, therefore, a public good, and as such it will not be provided in the right amount by an entirely free market economy.

THE PROBLEM OF PUBLIC GOODS IN A FREE MARKET

The explanation of why a free market cannot provide the right quantity of a public good will take the form of an allegory.

Consider several households living on a cul-de-sac in an area where snowfall is heavy. At the beginning of each winter, each household wants to ensure that some arrangement is made to have the cul-de-sac plowed whenever the snowfall is heavy. Each household benefits from whatever plowing is done but may differ with the others on when to plow. One resident may want the cul-de-sac plowed whenever two inches or more of snow falls. His neighbor who has purchased a four-wheel-drive vehicle will want considerably less plowing.

---

1. Another way to equalize income and well-being is to give money to some people. Many object to giving money, however, because doles decrease the recipient's self-respect and reduce his incentives to engage in productive activities.

Suppose that the households do not collaborate and that no resident takes the others' expected behavior into account in deciding how much plowing to arrange for. Each household contracts for a certain amount of plowing. Some contract for plowing whenever a little snow falls. Others contract for plowing only when the snowfall is heavy. The result is that when a heavy snow falls, several plows arrive to clear the cul-de-sac. Clearly this is inefficient.

Consider another possibility. Suppose that the residents still do not collaborate but that each takes the others' expected behavior into account. Each reasons, "The others are likely to arrange for plowing and therefore I don't have to bother to make my own separate contract." Since everyone thinks this way, no one contracts for snow plowing, and the cul-de-sac is never plowed. This, too, is an inefficient outcome.

The solution would seem to be for the residents to get together before the winter and decide how much snow plowing to contract for and how to divide the cost. This does not always solve the problem, however. Consider what might happen at the meeting to decide when to plow. Those who want the least plowing are unwilling to contribute to the cost of having only two or three inches of snow cleared from the cul-de-sac. They want to divide the cost according to the amount of plowing each household wants, reasoning that those who want more frequent plowing should pay more. Since each resident knows that his cost share depends on how much plowing he asks for, he has an incentive to ask for a little less plowing than he actually wants. He reasons, "Asking for less than I want will have very little effect on how much plowing is actually done, but it will reduce my share of the cost." Because each household has this incentive to ask for a little less plowing than he actually wants, the decision arrived at the residents' meeting likely will call for an inefficiently small amount of plowing.

This allegory illustrates two generally accepted assertions regarding the allocation of public goods: First, decentralized decisionmaking about public goods—that is, market allocations—will result in either too much or too little of the public good being provided. Second, even with centralized allocation of the good, it is difficult to determine how much of the good to provide.

Relating this allegory to the government's role in economic allocation, we may conclude that the complexity of a market economy, with its hundreds of thousands of commodities and millions of firms and households, makes government intervention an extremely difficult undertaking. Furthermore, once the government decides to intervene in the market allocation of a particular good or service, the difficulty of ascertaining the right level of provision suggests that the government probably will err in its allocation. At the same time, people may be worse off without government intervention. From the point of view of economic theory, a strong case must be made for intervention in the allocation of a good such as education before the delicate procedures of defining the right role for government are undertaken.

FACTORS COMPLICATING GOVERNMENT INTERVENTION IN THE ALLOCATION OF EDUCATION

The government's role in the allocation of education is complicated by the nature of education as a private as well as a public good. As noted above, such outcomes as general literacy, shared norms, and wealth redistribution make education a typical public good. At the same time, education is a private good to the extent that the attention that each individual receives in a classroom diminishes the amount of attention that the teacher can give to others. It is a private good also to the extent that a portion of the benefits of the schooling that each person receives is enjoyed by the individual himself and does not generate any public good. Specifically, by improving the individual's work skills, education enables him to earn a better living and also may improve the quality of his life.

The government's role is further complicated by the fact that the case for its intervention in education markets is a matter of judgment and individual preferences for education vary tremendously.

At one extreme, some people, given their social values, may find the arguments for intervention completely convincing, may believe that providing every citizen with a four-year college education at public expense will generate highly valuable social benefits, and therefore may support a high level of government involvement in the allocation of educational services. At the other end of the spectrum of opinion, some may place a low valuation on the public goods generated by widespread education, accept the distribution of income as it is, and therefore reject any government involvement in the education sector.

Others may accept the case for government intervention as a source of efficiency but argue that the public benefits of widespread education are exhausted at fairly low average levels of schooling. They might value, for example, the benefits of widespread literacy and therefore favor government involvement in elementary education, but argue that all of the benefits of higher education accrue to the individual who receives it. Still others may value public elementary and secondary education on efficiency grounds but view government involvement in higher education as valuable only as a redistributive device.

Our society has decided that widespread elementary and secondary education is a sufficiently important public good to justify some governmental action to allocate it. The problem then becomes one of determining exactly how much education each individual should receive.

DETERMINING THE OPTIMAL DISTRIBUTION OF EDUCATION

Economists have investigated two general approaches to determining the optimal allocation of education: the "social welfare approach" and the "local choice approach." Of course, neither approach can define exactly the optimal distribution of education. Both, however, through the analysis of economic models, suggest the kinds of empirical, theoretical, and value judgments that must be made in the process of determining the optimum.

The two approaches differ in the way they view the nature of education as a commodity. The social welfare approach focuses on education as a public good and analyzes the way in which a centralized government would allocate schooling. The local choice approach views education essentially as a private good but recognizes the fact that in the United States this particular private good happens to be allocated by public institutions, namely, local school districts.

The Social Welfare Approach

The social welfare approach begins with a hypothetical social welfare function—a mathematical statement representing certain specific social values. Under this approach we ask how much education each individual should receive regardless of how much he or she would choose to receive. A simple example (Arrow 1971) illustrates the approach.

Suppose that the social welfare function values only (1) aggregate economic well-being (i.e., the total quantity of goods and services produced) and (2) equality of well-being among the population. Different social welfare functions may place different relative values on aggregate well-being and its distribution. The distribution of noneducational factors of production among the population is assumed to be given. People sell their labor and receive income. The laborer's productivity determines his wage. More highly skilled, and therefore more productive, workers receive higher wages. Their income is higher, and it is assumed that they will be happier. Education increases people's skills and therefore the income that they receive.

The analysis of this model suggests two considerations that must be taken into account before we can identify the optimal quantity of education that each person ought to receive: how much any given amount of education increases any given individual's productivity and how much we value equality of economic outcomes.

A given quantity of education may increase the productivity of individuals with high innate ability[2] to earn income more than it would increase the productivity of people of low ability. That is, the total output of goods and services may increase more if a person of high ability receives an additional year of schooling, or schooling of a higher quality, than if a person of low ability receives the same additional schooling .Of course, the opposite may be true: Schooling may increase the productivity of low-ability people more than it increases the productivity of high-ability people.

Suppose that maximizing the total value of goods and services produced were the only objective. The sole criterion for allocating educational services then would be the degree to which increments of schooling improved each individual's productivity.[3] Given the as-

2. The term "ability," used here in a special, highly simplified sense, refers only to the ability to earn income, that is, the ability to be highly productive on a job. Furthermore, the term assumes that only one kind of productive ability exists. This assumption is obviously an oversimplification, because the ability to repair a car, for example, differs from the ability to play the piano. The results would be essentially the same even if the model were built around a variety of abilities.

3. If maximizing output were the only objective of allocating education, the government would have little reason to intervene. If wages were paid in proportion to productivity, each individual would have an incentive to buy just the amount of education that would maximize his contribution to aggregate productivity. The only reason for government involvement, given the sole objective of maximizing the value of output, would be that individuals were *not* paid in proportion to their productivity.

sumed social welfare function, if high-ability people benefited more in terms of eventual productivity than low-ability people, the distribution of educational services would be elitist. If equal increments of education benefited everyone equally, regardless of innate ability, the distribution would be egalitarian. If low-ability people benefited more, the distribution would be compensatory.

Maximizing the gross value of economic outputs is not, however, the only social welfare objective of the allocation of educational resources: The equity of the allocation is also an important goal and is the second consideration that influences the optimal allocation. This criterion usually is identified with the value of a fairly equal distribution of incomes by assuming that well-being and income are closely and positively related. If we provide educational services to people whose innate ability to earn income is high, we will be increasing the eventual incomes of people who would have received relatively high wages in any event. Hence, the resulting distribution of income will be more unequal than it would have been had we not allocated educational services in this way. If, on the other hand, we assign relatively greater educational resources to low-ability people, the allocation of education will tend to equalize the income distribution.

The identification of the optimal allocation of educational services among individuals in this model thus resolves itself into two questions:

1. Does schooling tend to increase the productivity of high-ability people more or less than that of low-ability people?
2. How much do we value any degree of equalization of income distribution?

Although this simple analysis does not completely define the optimal allocation of educational resources, it suggests several important observations about what such an allocation might look like. First, the optimal allocation probably will assign different levels of educational resources to different pupils. The pattern of productivity increases produced by schooling and the social value of redistribution are unlikely to dictate exactly equal expenditures. In the most likely outcomes, the level of educational services will either increase slightly as the individual's ability to earn income increases or decrease slightly with ability.

Second, the allocation of educational resources that maximize social welfare clearly ignores the individual's age, sex, race, and residence.

All that matters in this allocation is how productive the individual is likely to be, given any level of schooling, and how much we value improvements in the well-being of the individual. Of course, a social welfare function that values redistribution from one age group to another, from men to women, from whites to blacks, or from people living in one part of the country to people living in another part of the country can be defined. However, when the social welfare function ignores age, sex, race, and residence, the allocation of resources also will ignore them.

Finally, this model of social welfare maximization identifies the possibilities for conflict between output maximization and equity. If the allocation of schooling that maximizes output also tends to equalize the distribution of income—that is, if, in terms of productivity, low-ability people benefit more than high-ability people from the education they receive—there is no conflict. The conflict arises if society values redistribution but also finds that people with higher ability benefit more from education. In this case, whether educational allocations increase or decrease with native ability will depend on the answers to the two questions asked above.

This model can be constructed and analyzed to account for sources of income inequality, such as differences in ability, racial discrimination, differences in preferences for leisure, and even luck. In general, the allocation of education will follow the structure of the social welfare function and the assumptions that are made about the sources of inequality.

The social welfare approach might have descriptive validity in a country where educational financing was completely centralized. Students would be assigned to specific educational programs according to native ability or other factors that generate inequality. The distribution of services would be either elitist or compensatory, depending on the relationship between education and productivity and on the value of redistribution. A governmental social welfare function—say, that of the minister of education—would determine the optimal allocation.

The social welfare approach does not necessarily require the central government to produce the education that people receive. A system of subsidies or vouchers could be used to induce individuals to purchase education from private providers. Likewise, a system of intragovernmental grants and regulations could induce school districts to provide the optimal allocation.

The Local Choice Approach

The United States does not allocate educational resources according to a social welfare function. Rather, through mutual interaction, a complex set of institutions generates an allocation of educational resources among individuals. The institutions include state governments, the federal Department of Education, local school districts, private schools and associations, and other interested professional and lay groups. Local education authorities (LEAs) allocate available resources among the students who live within their jurisdiction and choose to attend the public schools. The aggregate resources available to the LEAs are determined in large part by the willingness of school district residents to tax themselves to support education. Other revenues come in the form of intergovernmental grants from state or federal agencies.

The local choice approach to the allocation of educational resources takes this institutional agreement as given. The simplest local choice models assume that different school districts may spend different average amounts per pupil and allocate available resources among pupils according to different decision rules. The models assume also that households differ only in the subjective values they place on education: that some families desire high levels of educational services for their children and that others are satisfied with less. In other words, the simplest local choice models ignore other differences among households—such as income. As the models become more complex, they drop these unrealistic assumptions and analyze how such differences affect the allocation of education.

This combination of assumptions—that all pupils in a school district must share the same aggregate revenues and that families differ only in the amount and quality of education they want—generates a fundamental efficiency problem. People with different subjective valuations of education must under these assumptions consume similar quantities. A simple model illustrates the inefficiency inherent in such a situation.

Suppose that there are equal numbers of two types of people: type H people, who are willing to pay for a high level of educational services, and type L people, who are unwilling to pay as much for schooling as type H. Suppose further that both types of people must live in a single school district, one that collects identical amounts of tax revenue from each household and spends an equal amount on each child in the district. Finally, assume that a central authority seeking to please local residents decides the level of taxes and services provided in the district.

Since the population is equally divided among the two types, the level of services might lie exactly halfway between the quantity desired by type H people and that wanted by type L. Clearly this distribution is inefficient. Type H people are receiving less education than they want and are willing to pay for, and type L people are paying for more than they want. If the district could be divided into two parts, segregating type Ls and type Hs and providing two different levels of educational services at two different tax rates, everyone would be better off, and no one would be worse off.

This solution of the efficiency problem involved in the local choice model suggests the widely discussed theory of local choice proposed by Charles Tiebout (1956). Tiebout argues that if the number of communities is large, the inefficiency associated with local choice will be reduced. According to Tiebout, if there are as many communities as there are types of people, everyone will be able to consume the quantity of local public services that he wants and is willing to pay for.

For the Tiebout model of local public choice to work, however, each household must be able to choose among a large number of school districts, each offering a different level of services. In fact, few households have access to as wide a variety of options as Tiebout suggests. People living in small metropolitan areas may have only one or two school districts from which to choose. Even in large metropolitan areas, work-place locations, economic constraints, racial discrimination, zoning laws, and other factors may confine the choices reasonably available to the typical household to a small number of school districts. It is uncertain, therefore, that the Tiebout mechanism actually results in an efficient allocation of educational services.

The local choice model, like the social welfare approach, does suggest some general characteristics of an efficient allocation of educational services. First, to the extent that households differ in their taste for education, the efficient allocation will be characterized by different quantities of education received by different pupils. Changes in school finance institutions that increase the choices available to the typical household are therefore likely to increase the overall efficiency of the allocation.

Second, as the analysis of the Tiebout model illustrates, allocative efficiency may be reduced when educational choices and residential location choices depend on each other. Because of the way school finance institutions operate in the United States, a household must live in a certain community in order to consume a given quantity of education.[4]. Educational preferences therefore influence residential choices, and, conversely, the choice of residence determines the amount of education that will be available. Most households wind up choosing neither the quantity of educational services nor the residential location they would have chosen were the two decisions not tied together. The result is a loss of efficiency. People might be better off if some way could be found for them to be able to consume just the quantity of education and just the residential location they want and can afford.

Reconciling the Two Approaches

The social welfare and local choice approaches provide two different ways of thinking about the optimal allocation of educational services among students. The social welfare approach distributes services among students in accordance with a social welfare function. The education each child receives is determined jointly by the values inherent in the social welfare function, the relationship between native ability and the productivity returns to educational investment, and the child's individual abilities. The local choice approach takes the institution of school districts as given. The education a child receives is determined by the services provided in the district in which the child lives. Residential decisions, in turn, are determined in part by the household's taste for education but also by work-place location, household income, racial discrimination, zoning laws, and many other factors.

These two approaches will, in general, result in very different allocations of educational services among children. Households are unlikely to arrange themselves in school districts in such a way that expenditures on each child will maximize anyone's social welfare

4. The choice of private schooling would remove some restrictions on the choice of residence, but private schooling involves essentially paying for education twice, once as tuition and once as local taxes.

function. On the other hand, a local choice model, in which all local educational services are paid for with local revenues, will not guarantee that the public benefits associated with education, literacy, shared norms, redistribution, and so on will be produced in the right quantities.

Legislatures and school finance analysts in the United States have suggested a number of ways to reconcile these two approaches. Higher levels of government can regulate the behavior of local school districts, dictating certain levels of services and the distribution of those services among pupils within the district. Intergovernmental grant mechanisms can supplement local resources. Expenditure limitations can help ensure that the distribution of expenditures among children does not deviate far from the social welfare ideal. Part Two of this study investigates the operation of these policy instruments in much greater detail.

Even with this array of mechanisms, however, reconciling the two approaches to the allocation of educational resources may still be impossible. The fundamental problem remains. The local choice approach is driven by the subjective preferences of households. The social welfare approach is driven by some objective understanding of the economic impact of education on aggregate productivity and aggregate distributional equity. As long as some individual choice is allowed, the allocation of education is unlikely to maximize social welfare. This tension is inherent in our federal system. The history of school finance in the twentieth century reveals a series of attempts to reconcile social norms and local choice. No school finance system can entirely eliminate the conflict, but a system based on a better understanding of how the two approaches work is likely to come closer to reconciling these approaches than a system that is not. In Chapter 3, we turn to a closer analysis of how local choice mechanisms generate the observed allocation of educational services.

SUMMARY

Public goods will not be allocated efficiently by the decentralized decisionmaking of the consumers and firms. Each household benefits by the entire amount of the public good provided, regardless of how much of the public good that particular household pays for. No household, therefore, has an incentive to pay for any of the public good, because it expects to benefit by the purchases of other households. Because no household has an incentive to pay, none of the public good will be purchased—an inefficient outcome. Some centralized decisionmaker is called for.

Education generates public goods. Public safety is enhanced by generalized literacy. The shared norms inculcated by public schooling are a requisite of social cohesion. Certain distribution of education services among children can lead to more nearly equal distributions of well-being among households.

Education is also a private good to the extent that many of the benefits of education are enjoyed only by the individual who receives the schooling.

Corresponding to these two aspects of education as an economic good (i.e., its public and private aspects) are two approaches to identifying the optimal allocation of education among individuals. The social welfare approach begins with an explicit set of social values and some understanding of how education leads to economic outcomes. The optimal allocation of education is the one that leads to the most valued set of outcomes. The local choice approach views education as essentially a private good. As such, education will best be allocated if each household consumes only the quantity of education it wants and can afford. If the institution of local school districts is accepted as unilaterally given, the local choice approach suggests that the more choices individual households have available to them, the more efficient the allocation of education will be. This analysis argues for a system of many small school districts, each offering different kinds and quantities of education.

The two approaches may lead to very different allocations of education among individuals. One of the central problems faced by school finance analysts and policymakers is to devise ways of reconciling these approaches.

3 THE PREDICTIVE THEORY OF EDUCATIONAL EXPENDITURES

This chapter reviews the economic theory of educational expenditures. It first identifies the institutional and behavioral factors that generate differences in spending per pupil among school districts in the United States and develops hypotheses about whether each factor increases or decreases spending per pupil. It then illustrates the application of econometric techniques to add quantitative content to the qualitative effects identified.

Qualitative and quantitative analysis of school district expenditures can be used to influence education policy. If we know which factors affect school district spending and to what extent, we then can call on policymakers to manipulate the factors under their control to change the pattern. The process of discovering the determinants of school district spending also provides information about how much different types of households value educational services. Knowing this, we can estimate the degree to which households will subjectively benefit or suffer from any given change in school finance patterns.

Partial equilibrium analysis is the basic methodology. We want to estimate demand and supply curves for educational services and to find out how these curves change when we alter the institutional context in which expenditure decisions are made. To apply the tools of supply and demand analysis to the problem of educational spending, we will have to develop concepts of the quantity of educational services and the price of a unit of educational services, as well as a model of how school districts make choices. Armed with these concepts, with the data available on school district characteristics and spending, and with the techniques of economic analysis, we will be able to show how the factors that we identify determine the expenditure outcomes.

The type of analytical results that we seek are illustrated in Figure 3-1, which represents the configuration of supply and demand in two school districts. In this case, we want to know why the supply and demand curves for the two districts are in different positions and what changes in policy variables might bring the service levels of the two districts closer together or drive them further apart.

Figure 3–1. Supply of and demand for education in two school districts

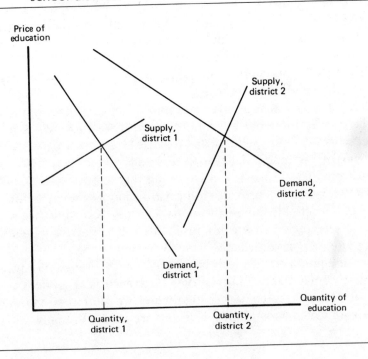

SELECTING A MODEL OF SCHOOL DISTRICT BEHAVIOR

The first task in analyzing school district behavior is to model it. Economic, social, and political models have been tried; the "median voter model" provides the most useful results.

Economic Models

Economists have developed and analyzed sophisticated models of individual consumer and firm behavior. A school district resembles a consumer in the sense that it decides how much education to purchase, but it is not an individual to the extent that the decisions of local educational authorities result from the complex interaction of many individual behaviors within the context of certain rules of process. A school district is also somewhat like a firm in that it produces and supplies educational services, but unlike a firm, it does not seek to maximize profits. Hence, the models of consumer and firm behavior do not apply to school districts.[1]

Organizational Behavior Models

Economists and specialists in related social sciences also have developed and analyzed several models of local government behavior. Viewing the administrative offices of a school district as a relatively autonomous organization, analysts can apply some of the findings of the sociological theory of bureaucracies (Gittell, Hollander, and Vincent 1970). Models of bureaucratic behavior describe the ways in which organizations respond to their environments. The characteristics of the school district—its population, its economic base, its location, and so on—constitute the environment in which its administrative bureaucracy operates. Although these models offer interesting insights into the essentially conservative nature of school

1. Some economists have attempted to develop firm-like models of school district behavior. This literature, collectively termed production function studies, goes beyond the subject matter of this study. Some of the implications of these studies will be discussed in Chapter 6.

district administrations, they fail to predict precise expenditure levels and therefore are of limited usefulness here.

Political Coalition Models

Some analytical work has been done on models of political coalition formation. School districts make decisions by political processes that seek to reconcile the different values held by the participants in the decisionmaking process. These participants include different classes of voters (rich and poor, with and without children, etc.), school district administrators, the school board, and school district employees.

Political models begin by identifying the interests of each participant group and positing some measure of the political power of each. The model isolates the possible winning coalitions of participants and predicts that expenditure outcomes must be consistent with the common interests of at least one of these possible winning coalitions. This class of models has a relatively high degree of descriptive validity. However, the political approach has not been applied to school district behavior because these models tend to become too complex to allow useful analysis (Salisbury 1970).[2]

THE MEDIAN VOTER MODEL

Economists most frequently use the median voter model to analyze school district behavior.[3] This model provides fairly precise predictions of expenditure levels, and its predictions approximate fairly closely the actual observed values. It has the further advantage of dealing with easily observable variables.

Assumptions of the Median Voter Model

The basic strategy of the median voter approach is to reduce the complex interactions that generate school district decisions to the

2. See Ordeshook (1978) for an illustration of the limited applicability of the political approach at this stage of its development.

3. The clearest development of this model is found in Bergstrom and Goodman (1973).

choice of a single consumer. The model allows us to assume that school districts act as if a single household—the household that is most typical of the community, that is, the median voter—made all decisions. In this, as in the case of many other economic models, the basic premise is that outcomes are generated as if the assumed behavior actually took place, regardless of the particular institutional structure of decisionmaking.

The model assumes first that the voters of a school district face a series of dichotomous choices of expenditure levels. For example, in a first election, voters would choose between, say, $1,500 per pupil per year and $2,000 per pupil per year. In a second election, they would choose between $1,600 and $1,750, and so on. Although no school district actually runs such a series of elections, the median voter model proposes that any decision mechanism that is driven by elections (budget elections, school tax levies, school board elections) will generate outcomes very close to those of the procedure described. Second, the model assumes that each voter is characterized by a preferred expenditure level and that the voter grows uniformly unhappier as expenditures decrease or increase from that level.

If these assumptions are granted, a single, specific level of expenditures will win an election against any other level of expenditures. This will be the level of expenditures preferred by the median voter; that is, half of the people in the district will prefer a higher level of expenditures and half will prefer a lower. Hence, if we can identify the median voter, we can model the behavior of a school district in exactly the same way that we model the behavior of individual consumers. The median voter model reduces the complexity of group behavior to the relative simplicity of individual household behavior.

Redefining Some School Finance Variables

To make the median voter model work, we first must define school finance variables, tax rates, and expenditure levels in terms that can be analyzed within the framework of consumer behavior models. In choosing which goods to buy, consumers take into account their disposable income, their tastes, and commodity prices. The median voter model assumes that the tastes and incomes of the consumer-voter are given, as are the prices of all goods except education. We are left with the problem of measuring the quantity and price of education.

We usually assume that it is possible to define a "unit of educational services," a hypothetical concept created solely to simplify the model. We assume further that one unit of educational services costs one dollar and that any quantity of educational services can be produced by a school district at a constant average cost of one dollar per unit. A district spending one million dollars a year is providing one million units of educational services.[4]

We assume also that each resident of the school district pays some share of the cost of each unit of educational services provided, called the "tax price" of educational services. The distribution of these shares is determined by the tax system of the district. For example, if the district's tax system dictates equal tax shares per resident household and if there are N resident households and no nonresident taxpayers, the share of the cost of each unit of educational services paid by each household will be $1/N$. More typically, since most school districts rely on property taxes, the share of each dollar of local revenues paid by each household is that household's share of total property value in the district.

This concept of tax price can be elaborated to take into account variations in the cost of educational inputs among districts and other factors. These complications will be discussed when we consider actual school finance institutions. At this point, we need only recognize that district financial decisions can be conceptualized within the framework of traditional theory of consumer demand.

Identifying the Median Voter

Analysts who use the median voter theory as the basis for empirical work generally identify the characteristics of the median voter as the median characteristics of residents of the school district. The income of the median voter is taken to be the median income of school district residents. The median voter's age is the median age of the residents. If more than half of the resident households contain school-age children, the median voter is assumed to have school-age children, and so on.

4. We do not need these simplifying assumptions connected with the unit of educational services. Instead, we can build a median voter model that more realistically defines educational services and the cost of providing them. Such models are complex but not intractably so. The predictions of these more realistic models are quite similar to the predictions of the simpler model.

Reducing the complex process of school district financial behavior to a straightforward application of consumer demand theory, we find that the same factors that influence any household consumption choice—prices, income, and taste—influence the spending behavior of the median voter.

The median voter model allows us to posit a number of hypotheses concerning the determinants of that spending behavior. These hypotheses rest on the assumption that the quantity of educational services per student is simply per student expenditure (recall that in the preceding subsection we defined a unit of educational services as what a school district could buy for one dollar).

The first hypothesis is based on the theory that, typically, when the price of a good rises, the quantity purchased decreases. We hypothesize, therefore, that

- The higher the tax price facing the median voter, the lower the expenditure per pupil.

The second hypothesis relates to the observation that as consumers' incomes rise, they purchase more goods. Therefore,

- The higher the median income in the community, the higher the expenditures per pupil.

The third hypothesis relates to the proportions of families in a community with children of school age. Typically, families with school-age children value local educational expenditures more than childless households do. Therefore,

- Expenditures per pupil in a district in which more than half of the households include school-age children will be higher than expenditures per pupil in a district in which fewer than half of the households include school-age children.

We may, in fact, expect to find that where the median voter is childless, school expenditures will be the minimum allowed by the state.

The fourth hypothesis involves the fact that consumers' tastes influence their consumption choices, and in this instance, consumers' taste for education is one of the most important factors. Although consumer tastes are difficult to observe, one might reasonably conclude that better educated people value education more than do poorly educated people. Thus,

● The higher the median level of education in a school district, the higher the expenditures per pupil.

Other taste variables, such as religion, ethnicity, and age, have been examined empirically in studies involving school expenditures, and equivalent hypotheses obviously can be stated for these variables as well.

The hypotheses as stated above are qualitative and directional. They do not as yet contain any assertion as to how much any particular variable might change per pupil spending. That is, they simply assert that when one variable goes up—with every variable other than the one of interest held constant—some other variable (in this case, school expenditures) goes up or down.

The techniques of econometric analysis, described in the next section, can be used to test these hypotheses and to add quantitative content to the model's predictions. We know that higher prices are associated with lower quantities, but the model does not tell us by how much. We must turn to econometrics to determine, for example, whether the median voter's choices are responsive or unresponsive to the tax price, that is, whether consumer demand for educational services is elastic or inelastic with respect to price. We know also that increases in median voter income are expected to shift the demand curve for educational services to the right, but we do not know by how much. When we ask these questions, we are also asking for a ranking in terms of importance of the factors that generate different levels of educational spending. As we shall see, the relative importance of these factors—price, income, and taste—is crucial to the design of school finance institutions that will work as we want them to.

Advantages and Disadvantages of the Median Voter Model

The chief advantage of the median voter model, aside from its relatively high predictive power and its conceptual simplicity, lies in its use of the concept of "tax price." Central (state) governments directly control the price of educational services. Matching grants from state governments and changes in tax systems can change tax prices and, depending on the price elasticity of demand, also can change expenditure behavior. The median voter model provides a method whereby a complex set of school finance institutions can be related to consumer and school district behavior.

The disadvantage of the model lies in the patent unreasonableness of some of the assumptions. The concept of a unit of educational services, an artifact of economic analysis, has no observable correlate. The choice process posited in the model, a series of dichotomous elections, does not describe the institutions of any known school district. Unfortunately, a model that offers the predictive power of the median voter model, its relative conceptual simplicity, and its usefulness for policy analytic purposes, but rests on a more realistic description of the ways in which choices are made, does not yet exist.

The Managerial Choice Extension of the Median Voter Model

A small number of economists (e.g., Barro 1974) have worked with what might be a more realistic extension of the median voter model. The decision process in the managerial choice model involves a single decisionmaker rather than a series of elections. The district superintendent, for example, decides the level of expenditures. The preferences, incomes, and tax shares of resident households influence the manager's choices, but other factors that may be of little concern to the median voter also influence managerial decisions. The superintendent may be more concerned with equity than the median voter is. He may value a rich educational program or high teacher salaries more than the median voter does.

If we could identify all of the objectives of a district manager and ascertain the priorities assigned to alternative objectives, we would be able to predict the effects of institutional changes on school district choice.

Two problems with the managerial choice model have led most analysts to seek elsewhere for their tool of choice. First, a manager who made choices at variance with the preferences of local voters probably would be replaced by one whose decisions better represented the preferences of the community. Second, managerial behavior is less well understood than consumer behavior. We are unable to posit a list of determinants of managerial behavior as concise and complete as prices, income, and taste. Empirical building under the managerial choice model is therefore likely to be ad hoc, and most social scientists prefer not to work with ad hoc models.

ECONOMETRIC METHODS

Our theory, derived from the median voter model described in the preceding section, tells us that X, Z, and W influence the value of Y. Here, Y is the "dependent variable" and X, Z, and W are the "independent variables." The relationships generated by the theory can be expressed as an equation relating the value of the dependent variable to the values of the independent variables:

$$Y = aX + bZ + cW$$

where a, b, and c are constant values, called "coefficients." The equation is an "econometric model," that is, an economic model translated into terms amenable to statistical treatment. We have two objectives: to estimate the values of a, b, and c and to determine how well our econometric model explains the differences we observe in the dependent variable.

A simple case using a pair of variables illustrates the objectives of econometrics. Suppose that we have collected and plotted variables E and T—for example, expenditures per pupil, E, and tax rates, T—for a sample of school districts. We might get a set of points, one for each district, like the set illustrated in Figure 3–2. Suppose further that we have developed a model which predicts that E and T will have the following algebraic relationship:

$$E = \alpha + \beta T$$

where α and β are constant.

To estimate values of coefficients α and β, we must find a single line lying as close as possible to all of the points in Figure 3–2. Such a line, AB, is depicted in Figure 3–3. Line AB can be represented as an equation in the form $E = a + bT$, with specific numerical values for a and b. If no other line lies as close to all the data points as AB, then a and b are the best possible estimates for α and β, respectively.

Figure 3–2.   Hypothetical data set on expenditures *E* versus tax rates *T* for a sample of school districts

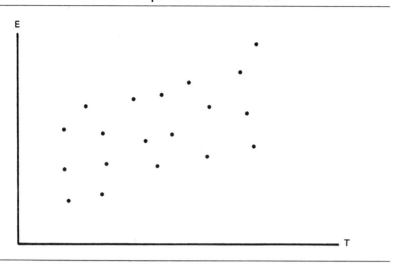

If we can find a line that lies close to all of the data points, as shown in Figure 3–4, we have a "good fit" of the data; that is, the model fits the data. If we are unable to find a line that lies close to all of the points, as shown in Figure 3–5, the model fits the data poorly.

Figure 3–3.   Fitting the data shown in Figure 3–2

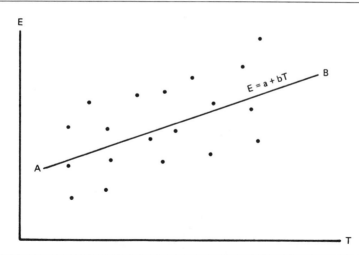

Figure 3–4.   Example of a good fit of model to data

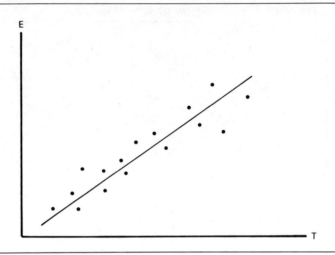

Figure 3–5.   Example of a poor fit of model to data

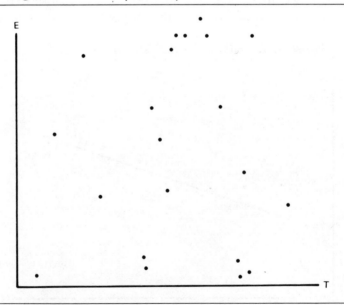

Econometric Analysis

Econometric analysis begins with data on the values of Y, X, Z, and W. For example, we might have data on expenditures per pupil for a sample of school districts (Y), along with census data on the median income of voters (X), their median level of education (Z), and local public finance data that would allow us to compute the tax price (W). We want to estimate a, the effect of differences in median income on district expenditures; b, the effect of differences in median educational levels; and c, the effect of differences in the tax price. Furthermore, we want to know how well these three independent variables, taken separately and together, explain differences in expenditures per pupil among school districts.

The values of a, b, and c can be estimated by applying econometric computational techniques to these data. Estimated values of coefficients are usually represented by A, B, and C. To compute the "estimated," or "fitted," or "predicted value" of the dependent variable, we add up the observed values of the independent variables, X, Z, and W, using the estimated coefficients, A, B, and C.

$$FY = AX + BZ + CW$$

The dependent variable for each observation (school district) in our sample now has two values: Y and FY, the "observed" value and the "predicted" value.

If we find that Y and FY, the actual and predicted values, are usually close together proportionally, we can say that our model is successful in explaining the variation in Y. If the values of Y and FY are frequently far apart proportionally, the model is less successful. This amounts to saying that the lines lying close to the data points in Figures 3–3 and 3–4 indicate a good fit or that the scattered data points in Figure 3–5 indicate a poor fit.

We can also evaluate the significance of individual coefficients.[5] We usually are interested in whether a specific coefficient—let us say C—differs significantly from zero. In other words, can we ascertain whether variable W exerts any influence at all on Y? We can answer

5. A coefficient is considered significant if there is a very good chance (usually 90 or 95 percent) that it differs from zero (or some other number).

this question by computing a predicted value of Y, which we will call FFY, assuming that coefficient C is equal to zero.

$$FFY = AX + BY + 0$$

The dependent variable for each school district now has three values: Y, FY, and FFY. We already have compared Y and FY to see how close together they usually are. Now we compare Y and FFY. If Y and FFY are usually as close together as Y and FY, then the variable W is not an important factor in determining Y, the coefficient C does not differ significantly from zero, and the inclusion of W and C does not help to predict values of Y. If, on the other hand, FY is usually quite close to Y, while FFY is frequently far off, we know that we can predict Y better by taking the effect of W into account and that, therefore, C differs significantly from zero.

Econometricians usually pay more attention to the significance of coefficients than to the overall fit of the entire equation. Our understanding of the causes of variation in a particular dependent variable often is limited, but our knowledge of the effect of one single determinant is fairly certain. Under these circumstances, we would expect to estimate an equation that has a fairly poor overall fit of the data but does have a significant coefficient on the well-understood term.

These tests of the statistical significance of coefficients also check the model's ability to explain differences in the dependent variable. Recall that the median voter model predicts that higher tax prices will be associated with lower expenditures per pupil. This means that coefficient C in our equation should be negative. If we found that the effect of tax price was zero, or, a fortiori, if we found that C was positive, we would know that the model's identification of school district choice with the traditional model of consumer behavior was mistaken. Fortunately, the hypothesis that the coefficient on tax price is less than zero has been supported by almost all of the empirical work on the median voter reported in the literature.[6] In other words, we find that we can explain variations in expenditures per pupil much better if we account for the negative effect of high tax prices than if we do not.

6. These studies are reviewed in Chapter 9.

Problems of Econometrics

Troublesome problems arise in econometric analysis when we attempt to estimate coefficients, such as a, b, and c, using real data. Some of these problems have been solved; others have yet to be solved or are inherently insoluble. Several examples of econometric problems follow.

Let us consider a somewhat more complicated model than the one described above, one involving "relationships between dependent variables." We continue to assume that the income of school district residents influences the expenditures per pupil, but we assume also that high-income people tend to choose to live in school districts where expenditures are high. In other words, our theory tells us that Y, expenditures per pupil, depends on, among other things, X, median resident income; it also tells us that X depends on, among other things, Y. This model can be expressed algebraically as two equations:

$$Y = aX + bY + cW$$
$$X = dY + eV$$

where d and e are new coefficients and V is another variable that influences residential choices. If this more complicated model is the true one, but if we estimate only the coefficients in the simpler equation, $Y = aX + bZ + cW$, without taking the second relationship into account, our estimates of a, b, and c will be wrong.

Techniques exist for dealing with simultaneous relationships between dependent variables, such as Y and X in this example, but few econometric analyses are able to take into account all of the possible simultaneous relationships among the variables under consideration. For example, some tenuous relationship may exist between W and X in addition to the relationship between Y and X. Our econometric model could be expanded to three equations, but only at the cost of more computation and only with data on some new variable. In using econometric analysis, we must judge which relationships among variables should be taken into account and which ones may safely be ignored. We ignore relationships at some risk and take them into account at some cost.

A second econometric problem involves "errors in variables." Suppose that our statistical sources are inadequate and that as a result our observation of, say, variable Z is inaccurate. If we fail to take this inaccuracy into account, our estimated coefficients will be wrong. Correcting for this problem again requires additional computation and more data and a judgment as to the importance of inaccurate data.

Yet another econometric problem, "colinearity among the right-hand variables," would arise when variables X and W, median income in a district and median education level of the residents, are such that when one is above average the other is almost always above average. In this case, it may be impossible to obtain precise estimates of the coefficients on these variables.

The extent of potential econometric problems and the expense of dealing with them call for several caveats:

1. Econometricians should make known which potential problems they have chosen to deal with and which they have chosen to ignore.
2. Consumers of econometric analysis should take account of the analyst's judgments and decide for themselves, first, whether the problems that the analyst ignored are important and, second, if the problems are in fact important, how much or how little faith to place in the findings.
3. Both analysts and consumers should beware the results of any single econometric study. Findings—for example, that higher tax prices are associated with lower expenditures per pupil—should be accepted only after several studies, using different techniques for different samples of observations, have reached similar conclusions.

SUMMARY

Economists most frequently use the median voter model to explain and predict differences in expenditures per pupil among school districts. Within the context of this model, school districts choose levels of expenditures per pupil as if a single household made the decision. That household is the median voter—the household with income, taste, and demographic characteristics most typical of the school district's population.

By identifying school district decision processes with the choices of an individual household, this model allows us to apply the insights of the theory of consumer behavior to the analysis of differences in spending per pupil among districts. Most important, the model highlights the role of prices in the decision process. The relevant price in the context of school district decisions is the tax price, the dollar amount an individual household must pay if expenditures per pupil in its school district are to increase by one dollar. Central (state) governments, it turns out, control this price variable. Analysis of the effects of tax price changes plays a major role in modeling the effects of school finance reform.

Econometric analysis translates the qualitative relationships predicted by economic theory into terms amenable to statistical treatment. The relationships generated by the median voter model are expressed as an algebraic statement, or econometric model, equating the value of a dependent variable Y to the values of the independent variables X, Z, and W, in the form $Y = aX + bZ + cW$, where a, b, c are constant values, called coefficients. Econometric computational techniques are applied to data on these variables to find the coefficient values. The estimated, fitted, or predicted value of the dependent variable is computed by adding up the observed values of the independent variables, using estimated coefficients. The coefficients enable us to ascertain the influence of the independent variables on the dependent variable and to test the fit of the model to the data.

4 THE THEORETICAL ANALYSIS OF TAXATION

This chapter introduces the economic theory of taxation. The theory derives from the same general unified theory that explains the working of many aspects of the economy. Although some of the conclusions of the economic analysis of taxation contradict intuition, these conclusions should be accepted because the theory as a whole works well.

The chapter begins with a discussion of the general criteria for evaluating alternative taxes: efficiency and equity. The second section presents the economic theory of tax incidence. The third section describes two general methods for determining who bears the burden of a given tax and demonstrates the application of incidence analysis— general equilibrium analysis and partial equilibrium analysis.

THE EVALUATION OF TAXES

Efficiency

There is no such thing as a perfectly good tax. A tax takes income away from a household and leaves the family with less to spend on the things it wants. In exchange, the government provides public services, which are valued by most households. A perfectly efficient tax and expenditure system would leave each household at least as well off after taxes have been collected and services provided as it would have been if no government activity had taken place. The utility lost by households when a tax is collected, however, almost always exceeds the utility gained when the public services are provided.

The difference between the value of the utility lost through taxation and the value of the tax revenues collected by the government is called the "excess burden" of the tax. Because this element of economic theory is an important aspect of school finance analysis, we will illustrate both discursively and by a special application of supply and demand curves how taxation leads to inefficiency in the form of an excess burden.

Recall that the prices of goods and services convey information to consumers and firms about the economic value of the resources they use. In deciding whether to buy an automobile, for example, a prospective consumer compares the subjective value that he will receive from that purchase with the price, which is the value that the market (representing society) places on the resources (factors of production) used to make the car. The consumer will buy the car only if the subjective value that he receives equals or exceeds the value that society places on the resources used to make the car. In this way, society's resources are used as efficiently as possible to create the greatest possible happiness for consumers. The price system conveys the necessary information.

Any tax (except a uniform or random lump-sum tax levied on all households) is simply the difference between the market price and the price that the consumer or firm must pay for the good. A tax drives a "wedge" between the price paid by the purchaser and the price received by the supplier. An excise tax on a commodity—say, a 10 percent tax on cigarettes—is the most obvious example, but most other taxes work in the same way. An income tax drives a wedge between the market price of labor (the before-tax wage) and the price that each laborer receives for his services (the after-tax wage). A property tax on land drives a wedge between the market price of land (the rent the user of the land pays to the landlord) and the after-tax rent that the landlord receives.

Once taxes have been introduced into the price system, the prices that determine household consumption decisions and firms' input choices cease to reflect the value that the market (or society) places on goods and services. When cars are taxed, for example, the prospective consumer no longer compares the social value of the resources used in automobile production with the subjective value that he expects to derive from the use of the car; instead, he equates the subjective value with the value of the resources plus the value of the associated tax. A tax, by distorting the equation of subjective and social values (an equation that results in an "efficient" use of society's resources as a source of subjective well-being), introduces some degree of "inefficiency."

The inefficiency introduced by taxes is graphically illustrated by the application of supply and demand curves (Harberger 1971). In this application, we view the demand curve in a slightly different way.

Consider a commodity, such as the *New York Times,* which everyone either buys one of or does not buy at all. Each consumer is willing to pay some price for a daily copy of the *New York Times.* The most avid reader may be willing to pay, say, $5 a day before forgoing the newspaper. The next most avid reader may be willing to pay $4.98, and so on down to the nonreader who might pay 1 cent for the newsprint.

Now suppose that the supply of the *New York Times* is perfectly elastic. In other words, assume that the Times Corporation can supply any number of copies at a constant price of 25 cents each. Anyone who is willing to pay 25 cents or more for a daily copy will do so. Furthermore, those who had been willing to pay more than 25 cents for a copy will pay only the same 25 cents that everyone else pays. It is reasonable to say, therefore, that the most avid *Times* reader, who would have paid $5 a copy, is enjoying what economists call a "surplus" of $4.75. He is purchasing something with a subjective value of $5 for a market price of only 25 cents. The next most avid consumer enjoys a surplus of $4.73, and so on down to the buyer whose subjective value of the *Times* is only 25 cents and who therefore enjoys no surplus.

Figure 4–1 illustrates this set of assumptions. It is as if the consumers of the *Times* were lined up along the demand curve in order of the price at which they would be willing to forgo consumption; the most avid reader is at the top. The surplus enjoyed by each consumer, the "consumer surplus," is measured by the distance between the demand curve and the price at which the good is sold. Thus, if the paper sells for 25 cents, distance AB represents the surplus received by the first consumer, distance CD the surplus of the second consumer, and so on. The aggregate consumer surplus derived from the sale of the *New York Times* at 25 cents a copy is proportional to the area of the triangle ABE, which represents the total benefit, or utility, derived by consumers from the production and exchange of this commodity.

Figure 4–1. Demand curve for goods selling at 25 and 35 cents

ABE = consumer surplus at 25 cents
AFG = consumer surplus at 35 cents
FHE = dead-weight loss (see below)

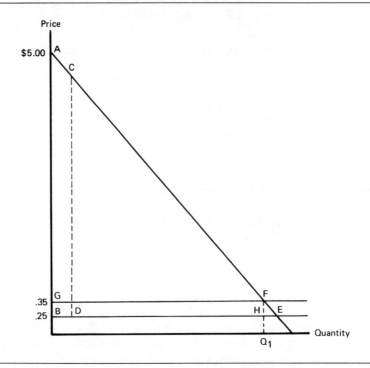

Suppose now that a tax is imposed on the sale of the *New York Times,* raising its price to consumers to, say, 35 cents. Fewer copies are sold, and aggregate consumer surplus is reduced to the area of the triangle *AFG*. The total government revenues equal the tax per copy, 10 cents, multiplied by the number of copies sold, *Q1*. The number of copies sold is proportional to the length of line segment *FG*, and the total government revenues are therefore proportional to the area of the rectangle *GFHB*.

Although a large part of the consumer surplus given up when the tax is imposed is transformed into government revenues that are used to provide valuable government services, another part is completely lost. The area of the triangle *FHE*, which constitutes part of the before-tax consumer surplus, is not collected as revenues; therefore it cannot be returned to consumers in the form of public services. The area of this triangle, representing the loss to both consumers and the government, is called "dead-weight loss."

A triangle of dead-weight loss appears when a tax is imposed, because some consumers who would buy the *New York Times* if its price represented the social value of the resources used to produce it no longer buy it. These consumers neither enjoy a consumer surplus nor pay taxes to the government, and the government collects that much less in revenues to be returned as valuable government services.

Although this example involves a commodity that everyone buys either one or none of, the analysis extends to all commodities. The triangle representing dead-weight loss appears under the demand curve whenever a commodity is taxed.

Based on this analysis, we can define the first evaluative criterion for taxation efficiency: A tax on commodity A is more efficient than a tax on commodity B if, when both taxes are used to raise equal revenues, the dead-weight loss associated with a tax on A is less than the dead-weight loss associated with a tax on B.

Commodities may differ in the degree to which taxation creates dead-weight loss; the relative elasticity of the demand for these commodities causes the difference. Figure 4–2 illustrates demand elasticity and dead-weight loss for two goods, the supply of which is assumed to be perfectly elastic. Two supply curves are shown, one at the initial price, P, and one at P plus the tax, $P + t$. The demand for commodity A is much less elastic than the demand for commodity B. The diagram shows the dead-weight loss associated with the tax on commodity A (triangle CEF) to be much lower than the loss associated with the tax on commodity B (CDF).

The example of Figure 4–2 reflects the general principle of efficient taxation: To minimize the overall inefficiency of taxation, the inelastically demanded good (in this case, A) should be taxed at a higher rate, and the elastically demanded good (B) should be taxed at a lower rate.

We so far have discussed the efficiency of taxation in terms of demand curves and consumer surplus, assuming that supply is perfectly elastic. If this assumption were true, it would mean that the producers of a taxed commodity bore none of the burden of taxation. The assumption is not true, however, and producers do bear a share of the tax burden.

Figure 4–2.   Demand elasticity and dead-weight loss
CEF = dead-weight loss from tax on commodity *A*
CDF = dead-weight loss from tax on commodity *B*

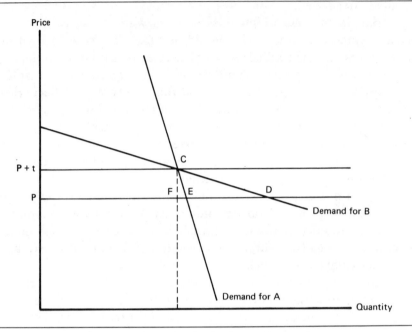

A producer, like a consumer, may enjoy a surplus as the result of the exchange of goods. "Producer surplus" is, in fact, the profits of the producing firms. Whenever a less-than-perfectly elastically supplied good is taxed, part of the producer surplus that would have been generated in the absence of taxation is transformed into government revenues and part disappears as a dead-weight loss. Dead-weight loss on the supply side is minimized when taxes are imposed on goods that are inelastically supplied.

Equity

To evaluate the comparative equity, or fairness, of alternative taxes, we first must determine who ought to bear the burden of taxation. We rely for this purpose on two widely accepted value judgments: the benefit principle and the ability-to-pay principle.

The "benefit principle" holds that those who benefit most from the provision of public goods should bear the burden of providing the revenues. According to this principle, the cost of supporting a public service that benefits a limited geographic area—for example, fire protection—should be paid by the residents of that geographic area. Likewise, because visitors to national parks benefit more from those parks than nonvisitors, but because even nonvisitors benefit to some extent from the park system, the cost of maintaining the parks ought to be divided somehow between the visitors and the nonvisitors. In this case, some combination of admission fees and support from general tax revenues appears to accord with the benefit principle.

According to the second general principle of fair taxation, tax burdens should vary directly with the taxpayer's "ability to pay." Based on this principle, households with higher incomes should pay higher taxes than households with lower incomes. The relationship between household tax burdens and household ability to pay may take the form of a progressive, a proportional, or a regressive tax. In the case of a progressive tax, the burden, measured as a proportion of the household's income, increases as income increases, so that people with higher income pay higher proportions of their income in taxes than people with lower income. With a proportional tax, the burden, again measured as a proportion of the household's income, remains constant for all income groups. A regressive tax places a higher relative burden on low-income households than on high-income households.

Good taxes based on the ability-to-pay principle of fair taxation exhibit both vertical equity and horizontal equity. A vertically equitable tax places a greater burden on households with a greater ability to pay. A horizontally equitable tax places an equal burden on all households with equal ability to pay. The horizontal equity criterion also may be interpreted to mean that differences in tax burdens among households should be based on characteristics relating to the ability to pay taxes, rather than on such criteria as race, taste, or geographic location. To the extent, however, that distinctions based on these criteria reflect differences in benefits derived, they would be justifiable criteria for taxation according to the benefit principle.

The Theory of Optimal Taxation

Both sets of criteria for good taxation—efficiency (minimization of excess burden) and equity—may be subsumed under the optimal taxation approach to evaluation. Models of optimal taxation begin with some general social welfare function that values increases in aggregate economic well-being and decreases in after-tax income inequality (Diamond and Mirrlees 1971; Atkinson and Stiglitz 1972). In such models, the government may be required to raise some predetermined level of revenues to finance public services, or it may collect taxes from some households to redistribute income to other households. Certain tax instruments—random taxation, lump-sum taxation, and taxes on leisure—are ruled out at the beginning. The problem, then, is to choose a set of tax rates on specific commodities or factors of production that raises the required revenues and maximizes social welfare.

The analysis of such models indicates that the optimal system of taxation

1. taxes elastically demanded commodities at relatively low rates and inelastically demanded commodities at relatively high rates;
2. taxes commodities that rich people buy at higher rates than commodities that poor people buy;
3. taxes goods that require a great deal of leisure time for their enjoyment at relatively high rates (to encourage people to work); and
4. avoids taxing factors of production (to insure that firms use the cost-minimizing combination of inputs).

Optimal taxation models, like all economic models, are based on some highly unrealistic assumptions—for example, that monopolies do not exist and that all consumers have identical tastes. Furthermore, none of the optimal taxation studies reported in the literature has analyzed optimal local, as opposed to federal, taxation. Because the structure of the federal taxation problem differs in several respects from the local problem, the results of the federal taxation studies should not be accepted uncritically in a discussion of school finance. Such analyses, however, do indicate some of the factors that ought to be taken into account in any evaluation of alternative tax systems and illustrate how issues of efficiency and equity can be combined into a single set of tax evaluation criteria.

THE INCIDENCE OF TAXATION

The "incidence of a tax" is the distribution of the burden of that tax among economic actors. One might say, for example, with regard to the incidence of the U.S. corporate income tax, that 75 percent of the burden is borne by owners of capital and 25 percent by consumers. "Incidence analysis" shows how the burden of the tax is distributed; that is, it identifies the household, or classes of households, whose well-being is reduced by the imposition of the tax.

In the basic model of production and exchange without taxation, consumers (households) sell factors of production and receive income. Firms buy factors of production at market prices and sell their outputs to consumers, again at market prices. Income and the prices of the goods that it wishes to buy determine each household's level of utility. The outcome of the process of production and exchange might therefore be represented by a list of the utility levels of all households.

When a set of taxes is imposed on the economy in the form of some tax rate for each commodity exchanged (many of the tax rates may be zero), consumers continue to earn income and firms continue to sell products. Because the government has changed some of the after-tax prices that influence firm and consumer behavior, the outcome will, in general, differ from what it was before the taxes were imposed. These outcomes also might be represented as a list of utility levels of all households, and the outcomes again would differ from what they were without taxes. A comparison of a household's utility before and after taxes would provide a measure of the burden of taxation on that household. The tax burdens of households under alternative tax systems also might be measured by comparing their levels of utility under each system.

This general model of production, exchange, and taxation does not, of course, provide a suitable framework for analyzing actual taxes. We do not know people's utility functions, nor are we able to build practical models to account for all of the exchange transactions, production decisions, and consumption choices which make up a real-world economy. The model merits analysis, nevertheless, because it serves as a basis for the more practical approaches to taxation discussed in subsequent chapters.

The model first of all illustrates the fundamental insight of incidence theory: The economic actor (firm or household) who pays the tax does not necessarily bear the burden of the tax.

The economic decisions that firms and households make after a tax is imposed differ from the decisions that they would make in the absence of taxation. The rational desire on the part of firms and households to minimize the burden imposed on them by the tax system motivates this change in behavior. Households that previously might have purchased large quantities of highly taxed goods instead consume less heavily taxed goods. Firms that might have used large quantities of highly taxed factors of production substitute other inputs. By shifting their economic choices, firms and households shift the burden of taxes that they might otherwise have borne to other economic actors.

Consider, for example, a tax on the purchase of new automobiles to be paid by the consumer. Once such a tax is imposed, some households that might otherwise have bought new cars now will buy either used cars or some other form of transportation. One result of the new tax, therefore, is a decrease in the demand for automobiles and, as a likely consequence, a decrease in the price automobile manufacturers receive for each car they sell from what it would have been absent the tax. Automobile manufacturers now sell fewer cars at a lower unit price and earn lower profits. The incomes of owners of these companies will, therefore, be lower than they might have been if the tax had not been imposed. Indeed, consumers probably will be worse off than they might have been if they were able to buy as many cars as they wanted at before-tax price. However, part of the burden of the tax will be passed back to the owners of the firms supplying the taxed good. Conversely, when the owners of firms are taxed, they usually are able to pass part of the burden of the tax on to other economic actors, for example, consumers and laborers.

The general model of production, exchange, and taxation illustrates an important limitation of applied incidence analysis. What we want to measure is the change in household well-being associated with the imposition of taxes. Because it is impossible to measure well-being, we must be satisfied with approximations of the ideal metric. Economists usually measure the change in a household's income brought about by the imposition of the tax. Furthermore, because it also is impossible to identify the effect of taxation on millions of individual households, economists usually do no more than analyze the effect of taxes on the incomes of classes of households, most commonly, consumers, laborers, and owners of capital. Economists attempt to compare the disposable, or after-tax, income of these groups with and without the tax under consideration. Finally, because owners of capital, as a matter of empirical observation, generally earn higher incomes than either consumers in general or owners of nothing more than their own labor services, economists usually assume that taxes that impose the greatest relative burden on owners of capital are the most progressive.

A set of simplifying and limiting assumptions—that income measures well-being, that owners of capital earn higher incomes, and that the quantities of factors of production are fixed—are implicit in any applied incidence analysis. When an economist says that under a given set of assumptions most of the burden of the tax is borne by owners of capital, he is claiming, in effect, that the price of all factors of production other than labor will be decreased by the tax and that the tax is therefore progressive.

The discussion of taxation in subsequent chapters is based on these assumptions; it should be noted, however, that not all capital owners fall into the category of those most able to bear the burden of taxation. Retired workers whose income depends on the earnings of a pension fund, for example, own capital, and taxes that reduce the price paid by firms for capital reduce the income of this class of households. Therefore, although a tax that places the greater burden on capital owners may be more progressive on average than a tax that bears more heavily on laborers and consumers, capital ownership is not a perfect measure of a household's ability to pay.

APPLIED INCIDENCE ANALYSIS

Because the perfectly general, multifirm, multihousehold model of production and exchange is too complicated to use in analyzing a particular tax, economists have developed simpler models of the effect of taxation. Three general approaches appear in the literature: two types of general equilibrium models—computational and algebraic—and partial equilibrium models.

General Equilibrium Models

The "computational model," the newest of the tax incidence models, most closely approximates the general model of production and exchange (Shoven and Whalley 1972; MacKinnon 1974). The computational model consists of a set of equations representing the tastes (utility functions) of consumers, the technologies (production functions) of firms, and the tax system. It can account for the interactions of a relatively large number of economic sectors, including several different types of firms (e.g., firms in the corporate and noncorporate sectors) with different production technologies (capital-intensive and labor-intensive). A computer solves the system of equations. The solution consists of either a description of the equilibrium allocation of all goods or a list of equilibrium prices of all goods. The equilibrium allocation is then used to compute the utility levels of each class of households. The system of equations is solved twice, once without and once with taxes. The utility levels of each class of consumers under the two tax regimes are then easily compared.

Although the computational approach might seem like the ideal tool for tax incidence analysis, it is limited severely by the data requirements. To specify a set of equations that can be solved as described, the researcher must build in a large number of facts. He is required to specify the precise characteristics of consumer taste and production technologies. The exact nature of the results of the model—the assignment of tax incidence—is frequently very sensitive to the particular characteristics of the utility and production functions. This difficulty can be mitigated by solving the equation system under several different sets of assumptions regarding taste and technology. This practice, however, often results in the finding that the incidence of taxation depends crucially on unknown, and frequently unknowable, facts. For this reason computational techniques have been used more as a check on other approaches to applied incidence analysis than as the method of first choice.

"Algebraic general equilibrium models" focus on the relationship between two or, at most, three sectors (Harberger 1962; McClure 1975). Unlike computational models, which require precise specification of consumer taste and production technology, algebraic models derive results that are true, given any of a wide variety of possible structures of consumer preferences and production technologies.

An example of the structure of a two-sector algebraic general equilibrium model illustrates these models and their use. Consider a metropolitan area consisting of a single central city, surrounded by a single suburban political jurisdiction. The area contains two classes of consumers: those who live in the central city and those who live in the suburbs. No one ever changes residence. Firms in the metropolitan area produce a single consumer good, buying labor services from the workers and renting land from landowners. All landowners live outside the metropolitan area. Consumers use their income to buy the single consumer good, the sale of which is taxed in the central city but not in the suburbs. Tax revenues are not used to provide public services in the metropolitan area. Firms can locate in either the central city or the suburbs.

These assumptions, along with the general assumptions that firms maximize profits, landlords maximize rents, and consumers maximize utility, can be expressed as algebraic equations. These equations can be solved. The solution tells us how the distribution of the burden of taxation among central city consumers, suburban consumers, central city landowners, and suburban landowners depends on the characteristics of consumer taste and production technology. One typical result is that if production technology is relatively labor-intensive, most of the burden of taxation will be borne by central city laborers, while if technology is land-intensive, a greater burden will be borne by landlords.

This example of a two-sector general equilibrium model typifies a wide variety of such models. Strong (unrealistic) assumptions are made so as to isolate the effect of one or two characteristics of production technology or taste on tax incidence. In this example, we isolated the effects of the labor- (or land-) intensiveness of production on tax incidence. A similar model might isolate the effects of consumer residential mobility, labor supply elasticity, or demand elasticity on the incidence of the tax in question. Models of this type, used frequently in the analysis of the incidence of the property tax, are discussed in Chapter 5.

Partial Equilibrium Models

An analysis of the effect of a tax on the market for a single commodity frequently provides an adequate approximation of the total effect of the tax. Recall that we used supply and demand diagrams in the section on the evaluation of taxes earlier in this chapter to illustrate the inefficiency inherent in all forms of commodity taxation. We use the same tool here to analyze the incidence of taxation.

The partial equilibrium analysis of taxation answers the basic question, which side of the market bears the burden of a tax? Or, to what extent does the tax reduce consumer surplus and producer profits? The usual method of analysis is to determine the effect of the tax on two prices: that paid by the consumer and that received by the producer per unit of the taxed good. If the after-tax price paid by consumers is the same as the before-tax price, then the entire burden of the tax falls on the producer. As the after-tax price paid by consumers rises, the burden shifts proportionally from the producer to the consumers.

The partial equilibrium analysis of taxation is illustrated in Figure 4–3. The curves D and S represent demand and supply in the absence of the tax; specifically, S indicates the net price that a firm must receive to be willing to supply a given quantity of the good.

Suppose that a per unit tax, to be paid by the producer, is imposed on the commodity represented in Figure 4–3. Now when the producer sells a unit of this commodity, he must pay $\$t$ to the government. To obtain, say, $\$P$ in after-tax revenues, he must receive $\$P + t$ from the consumer. The effect of the tax, therefore, is to shift the supply curve upward by a vertical distance equal to the amount of the

Figure 4–3.   Effect of per unit tax paid by producer

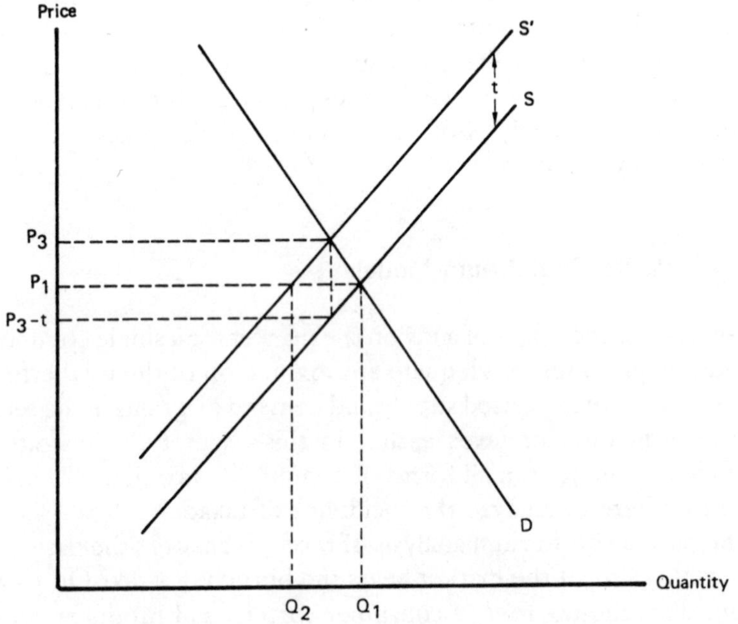

tax per unit. The new supply curve, S', shows how much the producer must now receive per unit to supply any given amount of the good.

The old equilibrium price and quantity, P_1 and Q_1, obviously cannot be sustained. If the producer receives P_1 per unit after the tax is imposed, he will be willing to supply only Q_2 units of the good, rather than the Q_1 units he had been supplying before the tax. The after-tax equilibrium lies at the intersection of the new supply curve, S', with the demand curve. At price P_3, the quantity demanded equals the quantity supplied, and the market is again in equilibrium.

Figure 4–3 shows the producer and consumer to share the burden of the tax almost equally. The price paid by the consumer has increased from P_1 to P_3. The price received by the producer has decreased by approximately the same amount, from P_1 to $P_3 - t$.

The tax burden is not always distributed as equally between the consumer and producer as it is in this case. Before we discuss the determinants of tax incidence, however, we will demonstrate that the

Figure 4–4.   Effect of per unit tax paid by consumer

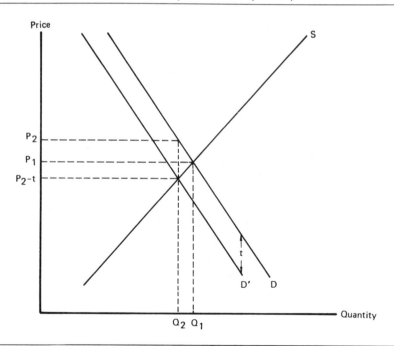

distribution of the tax burden is not determined by which side of the market—producer or consumer—actually pays the tax.

Figure 4–4 depicts the same before-tax market as Figure 4–3, except that now the consumer, rather than the producer, pays the tax of t to the government for each unit of the good purchased. The demand curve, D, represents the quantity consumers are willing to buy at any given price per unit. After the tax is imposed, however, when a consumer pays any price, P, per unit, the producer receives only $P - t$, and the government again gets the difference of t. The tax, therefore, shifts the demand curve downward by a vertical distance equal to the amount of the tax per unit.

The before-tax equilibrium, P_1 and Q_1, is no longer sustainable, because suppliers are unwilling to provide Q_1 units of the good if they receive only $P_1 - t$ per unit. The after-tax equilibrium lies at the intersection of S and the after-tax demand curve, D'. Consumers now pay P_2 per unit and purchase the quantity that they want, Q_2, at that price. The producer receives $P_2 - t$ per unit and supplies the quantity that maximizes his profits at that price. The quantity demanded equals the quantity supplied, and the market is therefore in equilibrium.

Superimposing Figure 4–4 on Figure 4–3, we see that the after-tax equilibrium prices to the consumer and producer are the same on both figures and that each side of the market bears the same portion of the burden on each figure. Thus, it makes no difference with respect to the incidence of a tax which side of the market actually pays the tax.

This conclusion simplifies discussing the determinants of tax incidence in a partial equilibrium context. We will analyze several paradigmatic cases, assuming simply that all taxes are paid by the producer, but knowing that the demonstrated results apply equally to taxes imposed on consumers.

The demand and supply curves in Figure 4–5 illustrate how the elasticity of supply and demand determine the incidence of taxation. *Case A* represents a perfectly elastic supply curve with a typical downward-sloping demand curve. Before the good in question was taxed, suppliers were willing to sell any quantity of it, as long as the price was at least P per unit. With the imposition of a tax, suppliers must receive an after-tax price of $P + t$ to be able to keep P for themselves. The new supply curve is represented by S', and the new equilibrium price is $P + t$ per unit. In other words, the price paid by consumers has gone up by the full amount of the tax. With a perfectly

Figure 4–5.   Paradigmatic incidence cases

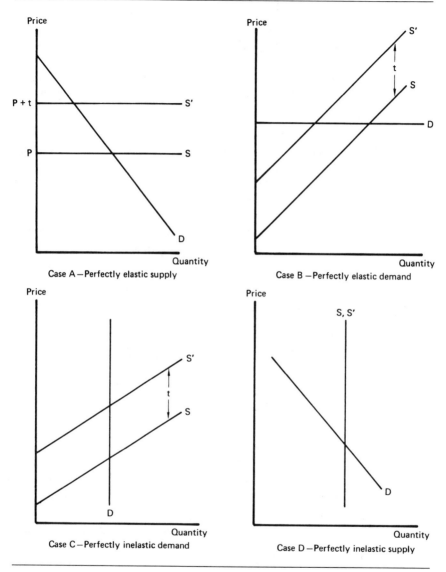

Case A—Perfectly elastic supply

Case B—Perfectly elastic demand

Case C—Perfectly inelastic demand

Case D—Perfectly inelastic supply

elastic supply, then, the entire burden of the tax is borne by consumers.

Case B is the mirror image of *Case A,* with perfectly elastic demand and somewhat inelastic supply. As before, the tax shifts the effective supply curve upward by a vertical distance proportional to the amount of the tax. In this case, however, consumers refuse to buy the good when the price to them rises above $P per unit. The price paid by consumers therefore remains the same, while the price received by producers decreases by the full amount of the tax. With a perfectly elastic demand, the entire burden of the tax falls on producers.

Case C illustrates a perfectly inelastic demand curve with a more elastic supply curve. Here consumers are unwilling or unable to substitute other forms of consumption for the taxed good. With a perfectly inelastic demand, consumers bear the full burden of the tax.

In *Case D,* the supply is perfectly inelastic: The quantity of the good available cannot change. The supply curve does not shift; consumers continue to pay the same price, but producers receive $t less per unit than they did before. With a perfectly inelastic supply, producers bear the full burden of the tax.

These figures illustrate a basic principle of incidence analysis: The largest proportion of the burden of any tax will be borne by the least elastic side of the market. This principle corresponds to a common sense notion. Inelasticity of supply or demand reflects inflexibility in economic behavior. The more inflexible side of the market is less able or willing to change its economic behavior so as to avoid the burden of taxation, and therefore it bears most of that burden. Although Figure 4–5 represents polar cases of perfectly elastic or perfectly inelastic supply or demand, the results also apply to intermediate cases. The burden of a tax is distributed according to the relative elasticities of supply and demand.

As always, partial equilibrium analysis presents an incomplete picture. We know, for example, that if the supply of a good is relatively inelastic, producers bear a large proportion of the burden of a tax on that good. We do not know, however, given only a partial equilibrium analysis, how the producer's burden is distributed among the owners of the firm, the laborers employed by the firm, or the landlords whose property may be rented by the firm. Likewise, we know that if demand is inelastic, consumers bear a large part of the burden. Therefore they have less income to spend on other things, and firms that would have supplied those other things can expect a decrease in revenue. The effects of taxation, especially of a good that consumes a large portion of a household's budget, clearly extend beyond the market for that good.

While partial equilibrium analysis is necessarily somewhat incomplete, the basic insight generated by that analysis is sound. The incidence analysis of any tax must answer a crucial empirical question: Is supply or demand more elastic? Econometrics, by providing empirical estimates of the supply and demand curves for the taxed good, can answer the question.

SUMMARY

Efficiency and equity are the two criteria for evaluating alternative taxes. The efficiency criterion dictates that inelastically demanded goods be taxed at higher rates than elastically demanded goods. When an elastically demanded good is taxed, much less of it is purchased. Consumers lose the benefit of that consumption, and the government collects no revenue from the lost sales. Taxation, to be efficient, should minimize this double loss of consumer well-being and government revenue by taxing inelastically demanded goods at relatively higher rates.

The equity criterion is associated with two principles of fair taxation. According to the benefit principle, those who benefit most by the provision of some government service should pay the most in taxes to support that service. The ability-to-pay principle says that those with a greater ability to pay should bear more of the tax burden than those with less ability to pay.

The incidence of a tax is the distribution of the burden of that tax among economic actors. Incidence analysis identifies the household, or type of household, whose well-being is reduced because the tax was imposed. Economists have devised several methodologies for determining which classes of households will bear the burden of a given tax.

General equilibrium incidence analysis shows how a tax will fall on broad classes of households—labor, capital owners, or consumers— depending on elasticities of demand for taxed and untaxed goods and the ability of firms to substitute different inputs.

Partial equilibrium incidence analysis uses supply and demand graphs to show that the burden of taxation of a single good will fall on consumers or producers of the good, depending not on who actually pays the tax but on the relative elasticities of supply and demand. To the extent that demand is inelastic, the burden will fall on consumers. To the extent that supply is inelastic, the burden will fall on producers. The side of the market that is relatively more flexible in its economic behavior will bear the smaller share of the burden.

5 THE CURRENT ANALYSIS OF THE PROPERTY TAX

The property tax constitutes the largest single source of revenues for public education in the United States. Recent school finance reforms have, to some extent, reduced this reliance on the property tax, but the tax remains a central concern of school finance analysts. Any change in school finance institutions necessarily involves changes in the property tax, and almost any change in property tax institutions necessarily affects school finance.

This chapter discusses the uniform and differential aspects of the property tax in the United States, who bears the burden of this tax, and the effects of zoning and income segregation on property tax incidence. The relationship between property taxes and the value of capital assets is analyzed in the final section of the chapter.

The property tax is an ad valorem tax, that is, a tax on the value of "real property," paid to the government by the owner of the property. Real property—also called real estate, capital, and capital assets—includes "land," "buildings," and "machines." A property owner's liability is a fixed percentage of the assessed value of the property, which is usually an approximation of its market value (the amount for which the owner could sell it), as determined by local assessors.[1]

1. Property value assessments tend to be somewhat inaccurate, but this inaccuracy does not bear directly on our discussion of school finance. In this chapter we treat the property tax as a fixed percentage of the actual market value of the property and refer to the process of real property assessment only as it applies to our discussion.

Economists agree that the traditional view of the property tax is too limited in several important respects and currently accept a "new" view that is, in fact, an extension and reinterpretation of the old view.[2] The discussion in this chapter is based on the new view.

The current analysis of the property tax stems from the observation that this tax, as administered in the United States, amounts to two separate taxes: a uniform tax and a differential tax. Almost all real property in the United States is taxed, and almost all jurisdictions levy some form of property tax. One way to ascertain the effects of the property tax is to analyze the incidence of a uniform, nationwide tax on all real property. The second way is to analyze the incidence of the portion of the tax that varies from place to place. The effects of these two taxes differ to the extent that the incidence of the uniform tax depends on the elasticity of the supply of capital and the incidence of the differential tax depends on the mobility of the economic actors.

The analysis of the property tax is easier to understand if we limit our discussion to taxes on business, rather than residential, property. The analyses of residential and business property taxation are, however, essentially identical.

THE UNIFORM TAX

The uniform, nationwide property tax is a tax on capital—land, buildings, machines, and so forth—paid by the owner of the capital. The incidence of this tax, like the incidence of all other taxes, is determined by the relative elasticities of supply and demand for the taxed good.

Economists generally assume that the aggregate supply of land, buildings, and machines is inelastic. This assumption is certainly true for the short run, because it would be impossible to alter quickly the total quantity of capital available. New construction and the production of new machines take time, and the total quantity of available land, even in the longest run, cannot be changed. If the supply of capital is perfectly inelastic, the burden of the uniform, nationwide property tax is borne by owners of capital. The income received by owners of land, buildings, and machines is reduced by an amount

2. A discussion of the economic analysis of the property tax, including a careful comparison of the new and old views, may be found in Henry J. Aaron's excellent *Who Pays the Property Tax? A New View* (1975).

equal to the revenue raised by the government. This point usually ends the analysis of the uniform property tax.

In the long run, however, the supply of capital may not be perfectly inelastic. The tax therefore may reduce the supply of capital, and part of the burden may be passed from capital owners to consumers.

Consumers' savings provide the source of new capital. Using some of the income that they might otherwise spend on current consumption, consumers invest in capital, usually by lending their money to intermediaries, such as banks, which then buy land, buildings, and machines or lend the money to other investors to buy land, buildings, and machines. In buying capital, consumers store income for future use. By reducing the income consumers may expect to receive from the sale or rental of their capital, taxes on capital reduce consumers' incentive to save.[3] The higher the uniform property tax rate, the less the incentive to save. If consumers save less, less capital is available than would be available had they saved more. Thus, a tax on capital may, in the long run, reduce the supply of capital.

If the supply of capital is, in fact, somewhat elastic, then part of the burden of the property tax will fall on those who purchase capital, namely, the firms. The owners of the firms, therefore, bear part of the burden of the property tax or, more likely, pass at least part of their share forward to their consumers or backward to the workers who sell their labor to the firms.

- The incidence of the uniform, nationwide property tax depends on the elasticity of the supply of capital, that is, on the sensitivity of consumer savings decisions to the after-tax income they receive for the use of the capital assets they own. Because most analysts assume that the supply of capital is relatively inelastic, they conclude that the burden falls on capital owners and therefore that the tax is progressive.

THE DIFFERENTIAL TAX

The differential property tax is a tax on capital, paid by the owners of the capital, in a specific location. Owners of capital in jurisdictions

---

3. This discussion holds all other determinants of savings decisions constant. Specifically, it ignores such factors as inflation, the income tax, and the position of the household in its life cycle. These other factors probably influence savings decisions much more than does the property tax. Nevertheless, this tax may have such an effect, and its absolute magnitude, if not its relative magnitude, may be substantial.

with high taxes must pay a higher percentage of the value of their real property to the government than owners of capital in low-tax jurisdictions. Again, the incidence of the tax depends on elasticities of supply and demand. To understand the effects of the tax in this case, however, we must revise somewhat our concept of elasticity. Instead of being concerned with the supply of or demand for capital in general, we now are interested in the market for capital in a particular location.

The Incidence of the Differential Tax on Business Property

If all capital were fixed in location for all time, the entire burden of local taxation would be borne by owners of capital in that location. In other words, suppose it were impossible to move machines, build new buildings, or allow old buildings to deteriorate. This would mean that the supply of capital to each location was perfectly inelastic. No matter what happened, the supply of capital in any given jurisdiction could not be changed, and capital owners therefore would bear the entire burden.

Furthermore, if all capital were fixed in location, the entire burden of local taxation would be borne by the capital owner when the tax was first imposed. Consider the owner of, say, a building in a specific jurisdiction. At some point in the past, this capital owner must have purchased his property at some price or constructed the building at some cost. The price originally paid for the building was determined by the rental income the owner expected to receive from that property. The higher the expected rental income, the higher the price of the property.[4] If the jurisdiction in which the property is located raises the local tax rate, the after-tax rental income that the property owner receives will be less than the pretax rental income. If the owner sells the building, the new price, based on a lower after-tax rental income, will be lower than the price he would have received if local taxes had remained at their previous level. The new owner, having purchased the property at the new, lower price, a price determined by the new after-tax rental income, therefore will not bear the burden of the tax.

Capital is not, however, completely immobile, and the entire burden of the differential tax may not be borne by owners of capital.

---

4. This relationship is presented more precisely in the final section of this chapter.

Although buildings do not usually move from place to place, they may be allowed to deteriorate and therefore to decrease in value over time. Owners of deteriorating property may use the money saved on maintenance costs to build new buildings elsewhere. By this process capital may move from place to place.

Capital is attracted to locations where it commands the highest price. A builder of an office building, for example, will choose a locality where the price per square foot of office space is highest, unless such factors as construction costs or the price of land are so high as to make the investment unprofitable. The after-tax price directs the location of new capital investments, since this is the price that the builder, or the landlord who buys the building, actually will receive.

To say that capital is mobile is to say that the supply of capital to any given location is somewhat elastic; therefore, part of the burden of differential property taxation may be borne by the firms in these locations. The higher the after-tax price builders or landlords receive in a specific place, the greater the quantity of capital that will locate there. If capital is elastically supplied to any given location, part of the burden of high differential taxation at that location will be passed on to those who demand the capital there, namely, firms.

The firms themselves also may be mobile. Firms will locate in the places where they can expect to earn the highest profits. If the price they must pay for the capital they use in production is higher in a given place, the cost of production there will be higher. Where the property tax rate is higher, the costs of production will be higher and profits will be lower. The firm therefore may choose to locate elsewhere unless some other determinants of the firm's level of profits make up for the disadvantage of a high cost of capital inputs. Unless the firm can sell its product at a higher price, or unless the cost of other inputs, labor, or land is lower, the firm will not locate where taxes are high.

Because both capital and firms may be mobile, the burden of differential property taxation must fall on the consumers of the firm's product, on the workers who supply labor to the firm, or on the landowners who rent their property to the firm. Which of these actors bears the ultimate burden of the tax again depends on the elasticity of supply and demand. If the demand for the firm's products is inelastic, the burden will be passed on to consumers. If the supply of labor to the firm is inelastic, the workers will bear the burden.

Inelasticity of supply and demand in this context have the same meaning as they have with respect to the supply of capital to a specific location. If consumers are mobile—that is if they can go elsewhere to buy the firm's products—demand for the output of firms in a specific location is elastic. If workers are mobile and can migrate fairly quickly to areas where they can obtain higher wages, the supply of labor to firms in a specific location is elastic, and workers therefore do not bear the burden of the differential tax.

If households, or some class of households, as consumers of goods produced by firms using highly taxed capital or as workers supplying labor to firms using highly taxed capital, are immobile, they will bear the burden of the tax. If all households, firms, and capital are highly mobile, the full burden of the tax will be borne by the owners of the only perfectly immobile factor of production: land.

- The incidence of the differential property tax depends on the mobility of the economic actors; those who are least mobile, that is, least able to escape high taxation by moving elsewhere, bear the burden. Because over the long run a substantial proportion of the burden of the differential tax is likely to fall on landowners, the tax is considered to be progressive.

The Incidence of the Differential Tax on Residential Property

The analysis of the effect of the differential can be extended to residents of the taxing jurisdiction, that is, to renters and homeowners. Owners of rental housing can be thought of as firms that supply housing. The capital used by these firms, the apartment house, is subject to taxation. If taxes in one location are higher than in another, landlords and builders will locate their buildings in the lower tax jurisdiction, unless, of course, the rents are high enough or the price of land low enough in the high-tax jurisdiction to make up for the difference in taxes. If the demand for rental housing in a specific location is inelastic—that is, if renter-occupants are immobile—the renters bear the burden of high local taxes. If the demand for rental units is elastic, then the burden of the tax is passed backward to landowners.

The differential property tax on owner-occupied housing raises the price a homeowner must pay to reside in a certain community. Everything else being equal, a potential buyer would prefer to buy a house in a low-tax rather than a high-tax jurisdiction. If potential buyers are free to choose among a large number of communities, each with a different local tax rate, then the demand for housing in each community will be highly elastic and the supplier of owner-occupied housing will bear the burden of the tax. The suppliers, or current owners, of houses in high-tax jurisdictions must reduce their selling prices below those of similiar houses in low-tax localities if they wish to sell. The current owner, therefore, bears a large part of the burden. If, however, when the current owner buys his house, he too is able to pass the burden of differential taxation backward, then it is the original owner of the property at the time the differential tax was imposed who bears the burden of the tax.[5]

If, on the other hand, the potential buyer's demand for a specific location is inelastic—if for some reason he is unwilling or unable to locate in a low-tax community—a larger part of the burden of differential taxation will fall on him.

The logic of these cases—business property, rental housing, and owner-occupied housing—is identical. The economic actors who are least flexible in their choice of locations, that is, who are least mobile, will bear the greatest burden of differential local taxation.

The Effect of Mobility on Incidence

The incidence of the differential property tax depends, then, on the mobility of the various economic actors, and the distribution of the burden obviously will differ from the short run to the long run. In the short run—say, for the first year or so after a locality increases its property tax rate—all economic actors are probably immobile. Because capital, the taxed factor, is immobile and therefore inelastically supplied to the locality, owners of capital located in the jurisdiction initially will bear the burden of the new tax.

In the long run, however, capital owners will respond to the new tax by moving their capital—reducing their investment in the higher tax locality and investing more heavily elsewhere. As the supply of capital is reduced in the jurisdiction, its price rises, and the burden of taxation is passed on by the firms that use the higher priced capital to consumers, workers, or landowners. Households that are unable to move in

5. This mechanism is discussed in greater detail in the final section of this chapter.

response to higher prices for consumer goods and lower wages will bear part of the burden.

In the very long run, enough households will have moved out and the demand for locally produced goods will have diminished enough so that the price charged for those goods will have dropped to the old, before-tax level. Likewise, outmigration will reduce the supply of labor, raising wages to the pretax level. Once all mobile factors have responded, the burden of the tax will fall on landowners.

What proportion of the total burden falls on each group of actors, and therefore the equity of the differential property tax, depends on the relative degrees of mobility. Given the current state of empirical knowledge of factor mobility, economists are unable to define a precise allocation of the burden of the differential property tax. They know, however, that people in the United States are highly mobile. The past three decades have witnessed one of the largest and fastest migrations of population in history, the movement of rural southern blacks to the urban north. Furthermore, according to the U.S. Census, the average household moves once every five years. Capital is also highly mobile, as witness the recent shift in investment from central cities to the suburbs and from the northeast to the south and west.

The Effect of Zoning and Income Segregation on Incidence

Bruce Hamilton (1976) pointed out a way in which the property tax might work to the disadvantage of low-income households. Assuming that all residents of a jurisdiction benefit equally from the public services provided by the local government, he reasons as follows. Because an individual's tax bill is proportional to the value of his property, richer households pay more in taxes than poorer households. The use of the property tax, therefore, necessarily involves a degree of intrajurisdictional income redistribution. Wealthier households pay more in taxes than it costs to provide their share of public services, while poorer households pay less. The rich, in effect, subsidize the poor's consumption of public services. The presence of low-income households, therefore, creates a burden on the wealthier taxpayers in a jurisdiction. This inherent redistribution associated with the property tax creates an incentive for those at the upper end of the local income distribution to try to discourage lower income households from moving into the community.

The institution of minimum lot size or single-family zoning, according to Hamilton, provides a mechanism by which wealthier households can effectively exclude lower income households from certain communities. This confluence of motive and opportunity has two effects. The first effect is a tendency toward income segregation. If all communities acted on the incentive to exclude potential residents with incomes below the current median of the community, then in equilibrium each community would consist only of households falling within some narrow range of incomes.

The second effect is the lack of an incentive to provide housing for the poorest households. If all communities failed to provide such housing, the supply of housing for very low-income households would be limited and these households would pay more for their housing. Furthermore, the residential mobility of low-income households would be reduced, and they would therefore bear a higher proportion of the burden of differential property taxes in the few communities in which they were able to live. Hamilton concludes, therefore, that the institution of zoning might add an element of regressivity of the property tax.

TAXES AND THE VALUE OF CAPITAL ASSETS

This chapter has discussed the nonquantitative determinants of the price of capital assets (land, buildings, and machines). The price, or value, of such an asset is determined by the income a potential buyer may expect to receive by renting this asset to a firm or, in the case of residential housing, to the household. The higher the expected stream of rental income, the higher the value of the asset. Property taxes, that is, taxes on capital income, reduce the net income an owner may expect to receive from that capital and therefore reduce the price a potential investor would be willing to pay for it.

Our understanding of this relationship, which is crucial to a general understanding of the incidence of the property tax, can be deepened by adding some quantitative content to this qualitative analysis. A more precise description of how the price of an asset is determined follows.

We begin with a simple problem. What amount would an investor have to deposit in a bank in order to be able to withdraw $100 per year for 10 years and have nothing left at the end? Since banks pay interest on deposits, the amount the investor would have to deposit would be less than 10 × $100 = $1,000. Exactly how much would he have to deposit?

To solve the problem, we divide it into ten separate problems and ask how much the investor would have to deposit now in order to withdraw $100 in one year, how much he would have to deposit now in order to withdraw $100 in two years, and so on.

The first question can be answered by solving a simple algebraic equation. We know that he will earn some rate of interest on his deposit, and we represent this rate by r. The interest rate on bank deposits is usually around 6 or 7 percent, so $r = 0.06, 0.07$, or something in that range. If he deposits $X in a bank account, by the end of one year he will have $X + rX = $X(1 + r)$. If he wants to withdraw $100 at the end of the year, he must deposit $X so that:

$$X(1 + r) = \$100$$

Therefore

$$X = \frac{\$100}{(1 + r)}$$

Now consider the second-year problem. If he deposits $X, he will have $X(1 + r)$ by the end of the first year and $X(1 + r) + X(1 + r)r = X(1 + r)(1 + r) = X(1 + r)^2$ by the end of the second year. Therefore, if he wants to withdraw $100 at the end of two years, he must deposit $X so that

$$X(1 + r)^2 = \$100$$

or

$$X = \frac{\$100}{(1 + r)^2}$$

By similar development, the amount that he must deposit in order to withdraw $100 in three years is

$$X = \frac{\$100}{(1 + r)^3}$$

and so on.

We now return to the original question of how much he would have to deposit initially in order to withdraw $100 per year for ten years. We simply add all of the individual amounts that he would have to deposit in order to withdraw $100 for each individual year. The initial deposit would have to be

$$\frac{\$100}{(1 + r)} + \frac{\$100}{(1 + r)^2} + \cdots + \frac{\$100}{(1 + r)^{10}} = V$$

V represents the "net present value" of a stream of ten annual payments of $100 each. Once we know r, we easily can compute V.

The same logic underlies the determination of net present value or the price of any capital asset that yields income. The interest rate, r, sometimes referred to as the rate of return or discount rate, will differ for different types of capital assets. Banks offer among the most reliable financial investments in our economy. Such investments as land, buildings, and corporate stocks yield less certain income streams. The more uncertain the income stream yielded by a capital asset—that is, the riskier the asset—the higher will be the interest rate used to determine the value of the asset. However, the algebra of the relationship between the income stream and the value of the asset is identical.

Suppose we have a capital asset (land, a building, a stock, or a bond) that is expected to yield $Y a year in rental income for a fifty-year period. The value of that asset will be

$$V = \frac{Y}{(1 + r)} + \frac{Y}{(1 + r)^2} + \cdots + \frac{Y}{(1 + r)^{50}}$$

A potential investor would be willing to pay $V for this hypothetical asset. Suppose that a tax of $T per year is imposed on the income yielded by this asset. What will be the effect of this tax on the value an investor would be willing to pay for this particular asset? Now, instead of $Y per year, the investor will receive $Y - T per year. A tax on a single asset, or on all of the assets located in a particular jurisdiction, will have little effect on the rate of return, or interest rate, earned by investors in general. Therefore, r will not change. The new value for the asset, V', can be computed according to the same formula:

$$V' = \frac{Y-T}{(1 + r)} + \frac{Y-T}{(1 + r)^2} + \cdots + \frac{Y-T}{(1 + r)^{50}}$$

This can be rewritten as:

$$V' = \left(\frac{Y}{(1 + r)} + \cdots + \frac{Y}{(1 + r)^{50}} \right) - \left(\frac{T}{(1 + r)} + \cdots + \frac{T}{(1 + r)^{50}} \right)$$

The term inside the rightmost set of parentheses of this last equation is the "net present value of the tax payment stream." It is equal, in other words, to the investment one would have to make in order to receive an income stream equal to the amount of the taxes due each year on the original asset.

Consider the situation of an investor who had bought the asset before the tax was imposed and paid V for it. Suppose the investor decides to sell the asset to someone else after the tax is imposed. The original owner will receive only V', rather than the V he originally paid for the asset. The difference between the price the original investor paid and the price he receives from the sale, $V - V'$, exactly equals the net present value of the tax payment stream.

Who then bears the burden of the tax? The new owner, who will pay the annual tax to the government, has purchased an asset that yields $Y - T$ a year at a price of V', exactly what any investor would be willing to pay for such an asset. The new owner, therefore, bears no burden. The original owner bears the entire burden in the form of a loss on his purchase and sale of the asset. The entire burden of the tax is borne by the owner of the asset at the time the tax is imposed.

This discussion refers only to the effect of taxes on specific capital assets or on some small proportion of the total capital available in the economy. It might apply, for example, to an increase in property taxes in a specific small jurisdiction. A general tax on all capital, such as the nationwide uniform property tax, would not have the same effect. A tax on all capital reduces the income yielded by each capital asset. A uniform tax on capital would reduce the net interest received by owners of bank accounts. A 50 percent tax on all capital income, for example, would reduce the net interest payment on bank accounts from 6 percent to 3 percent. In other words, our discussion of the effect of taxes on the values of specific capital assets refers to the effects of differential property taxes only. This general phenomenon—the effect of taxes on the value of capital assets—is referred to in the economic literature as the "capitalization" of property taxes.

SUMMARY

As we have seen, the property tax is subject to two separate analyses. The effect of the nationwide, uniform average property tax rate generally is assumed to reduce the incomes of owners of capital. This

25

Tue Oct 18 1994

WSU Dunbar Library
Col. Glenn Highway
Dayton, Ohio 45435
513-873-2525

A hold has been placed on the following item by the patron
listed below. Please pull this item and forward it to the
library location given below.

AUTHOR: Gurwitz, Aaron S
The economics of public school fina
CALL NO: LB2825 .G86 1982
BARCODE: 00013023348147
STATUS: CHECK SHELVES
Dunbar Stacks

P685(F94)
CHRISTOPHER M THOMAS
2070 HEWITT AVE
KETTERING OH 45440

conclusion is qualified somewhat by the consideration that if the income that capital owners receive from their investments is reduced, they may save less of their current income. A reduction in the quantity of available capital may result either in increases in the prices of outputs, especially those of firms that use large amounts of taxed capital inputs, or in reductions in the wages paid to workers. The importance of this qualification with respect to the long-run elasticity of the supply of capital is uncertain, and most economists appear to accept the conclusion that the burden of the nationwide average property tax falls on capital owners. If so, the tax is progressive, since capital owners, as a class, tend to be better off than those who have nothing to sell but their labor services.

The incidence of the differential property tax, the part of the tax that varies among locations, falls on the least mobile economic actors. In the short run, an increase in local taxes will affect those who pay the tax, the capital owners, because they cannot move their capital quickly. Over a longer period, capital can, in a sense, move from high-tax to low-tax jurisdictions. Once this has happened, the burden of high local taxes will fall on other economic actors—consumers or laborers. The least mobile will bear the burden for the longest time. Eventually all economic actors will have responded, leaving only the perfectly immobile landowners to bear the ultimate burden. The distribution of burdens will depend on how fast these adjustments take place. Over the long run, however, a substantial proportion of the burden is likely to fall on landowners, and the differential property tax too is considered progressive.

The conclusion that the property tax is essentially progressive, however, must be modified somewhat in light of Hamilton's analysis. To the extent that exclusive zoning is a major factor in determining the residential patterns of different income classes, part of the burden of the property tax may be borne by low-income households.

6 ECONOMIC THEORIES OF SCHOOL DISTRICT GOVERNANCE

Our discussion to this point had dealt with two school finance variables: expenditures and tax rates. This chapter goes one step beyond these variables to investigate how gross expenditures are transformed into educational services.[1]

School district managers turn expenditures into educational services, using the money made available to them by local taxpayers and state and federal aid to purchase educational inputs, including teacher services, materials, and buildings. In this sense, the behavior of school district managers is superficially analogous to that of the managers of private sector firms. The incentives that determine the behavior of school managers, however, differ from those influencing the choices of private sector managers. Furthermore, the output produced by school managers—education—differs in several important respects from the product produced by the paradigmatic private sector firm. For these reasons, the attempt to develop economic models of school district managerial behavior has been less successful than other attempts to apply economic theory to school finance questions. Nevertheless, some economists have tackled these issues, and their findings suggest some insights into how districts are and ought to be managed.

We begin by defining the role of the school district manager in economic terms—that is, we ask what it is that school district mana-

1. The step after this one, the investigation of how services are transformed into educational outcomes, is equally important, but far beyond the scope of this report.

gers attempt to maximize. In all of the economic models discussed so far, each actor's objectives are well-defined, at least in principle. Consumers maximize utility. Firms maximize profits. Governments maximize social welfare. The objectives of school district managers can be viewed in two different ways.

According to the normative theory of school district managerial behavior, because a school district is a government agency, its managers should attempt to maximize social welfare. Social welfare is again defined as some aggregation of individual household levels of well-being. In other words, the school district manager should act to make his clients, the residents of the school district, as well off as they can possibly be, given the total resources available to the community and the tastes of the residents.

A predictive theory of district managers' behavior might be built around an attempt to ascertain the objectives that actually inform managerial choices. School district managers are individuals with their own preferences and objectives. Some simply might want to maximize their own income; others may seek to increase the probability of being reelected or reappointed to their current jobs, or to rise in the hierarchy of the education profession, or to send a high percentage of their pupils to Ivy League schools.

A NORMATIVE THEORY OF MANAGERIAL BEHAVIOR

The environment of a school district manager consists of the district's clientele and the local markets for educational inputs. The clientele—the residents of the district and the firms located in the district—contribute to the financial support of district operations. Other sources of financial support are state and federal grants. Each resident of the district assigns some subjective value to education in general and to each specific output of the schools—basic skills, advanced skills, affective outcomes, and so on.

We assume that procedures—elections, for example—exist for translating these individual preferences into a social welfare function for the school district. We assume also that some other set of procedures, other elections possibly, determines the total financial resources available to the district manager.

The manager's job is to design an educational program that will produce the level and combination of outputs that maximizes local social welfare, given the total budget available. The educational program, in turn, consists of a set of educational inputs, including teachers, materials, and facilities.

These assumptions generate a model so complex that few normative insights can be derived from an analysis based only on these assumptions. To derive any prescriptions at all, we must begin by analyzing simpler models.

The first simplifications are radical assumptions: (1) that school districts produce a single output; (2) that district managers face a completely understood and certain production technology; and (3) that all educational inputs are supplied to districts at a constant price per unit (i.e., all factors of educational production are perfectly elastically supplied). After an analysis of this highly simplified model in this chapter, we will drop the first two assumptions in turn and discuss the ways in which the conclusions are changed by making the assumptions more realistic. We will drop the final assumption, that of a perfectly elastic supply of inputs, in Appendix A.

A district manager faced with a known technology, a set of input prices, and a fixed budget should attempt to choose the combination of inputs that will enable him to produce the highest level of output, given the fixed budget. Two considerations enter into the manager's decisions regarding how much of each input to use: the unit price of each input and the productivity of that input. This hypothetical manager will choose to use large quantities of the most productive and least expensive inputs. Inputs that are less productive and more expensive will be used more sparingly.

This simple prescription is complicated by two general characteristics assumed to be shared by all production technologies. First, we assume that the productivity of any given input is determined in part by the quantity of other inputs that are in use. We assume, for example, that the better the environment in which teachers work, the more productive they will be. In other words, the better the quality of the school building and the richer the available supply of materials, the higher the output produced by any given teaching staff. Second, we assume that the productivity of any single input, all other inputs being held constant, diminishes on the margin. In other words, the additional output produced by one more teacher will be greater if that teacher is added to a staff of 100 than if he is added to a staff of 1,000, all other inputs held constant.

These two assumptions taken together tell us that the optimal decisions for a school district manager will involve the use of a combination of inputs. It does not pay to spend all of the budget on teachers, for example, because each additional teacher hired produces a smaller increment of output than the previous teachers hired; at the same time, the productivity of all teachers is enhanced by investments in other inputs.

When we assume that the production technology is known, we really are assuming that the district manager knows all about these productivity relationships. He knows, for example, by how much output will be increased if, given some existing combination of inputs, the teaching staff, the quality of buildings, or the stock of equipment is increased by one unit. The normative result of this analysis is as follows: In choosing a combination of inputs, the school district manager should take into account the productivity and unit cost of each individual input, considered as part of a combination of other inputs.

Some of the assumptions used to derive this conclusion are patently unrealistic. However, the fundamental nature of the prescription remains the same when we drop the assumptions. Our notion of productivity must be revised somewhat when we change the assumptions, but the prescription—that we consider all inputs simultaneously and use a large quantity of inputs whose productivity is high relative to their unit cost—remains the same.

Let us drop the first radical assumption noted above: that school districts produce a single output. We know this to be false. Suppose, in fact, that districts produce multiple outputs and that the outputs are interdependent. The more of one output (e.g., reading test scores) a district produces, the easier it will be for the district to produce other outputs (e.g., effective skills). In deciding how much of a given input to use, we must take into account its productivity with respect to each of the outputs of the district taken together and the productivity relationships among the outputs themselves.

Consider, for example, the decision of a school district regarding the purchase of a computer-assisted reading program. We will want to know the cost of the system and the increase in reading and other tests scores that the program is expected to produce. We also will want to know the impact of improved reading skills on the production of other educational outputs. If we define productivity broadly enough to include all of direct and indirect effects of each input, as part of a combination of inputs, on all outputs, the prescription remains the same.

Now we drop the second assumption regarding the district manager's certain knowledge of the production technology. The manager is not completely ignorant of all productivity relationships but is more or less uncertain about the size of the increase in output produced by an increase in any given input. One possible prescription for managers faced with this kind of uncertainty would be to base input choices on his or her best guess as to the production relationships among inputs.

Such a conclusion, however, would ignore one important element of the social welfare function that the manager is attempting to maximize. Some input combinations might be characterized by more uncertainty than others. A new curricular program, for example, which looks highly productive in theory but is largely untried, might be rejected in favor of a more traditional approach that offers a smaller, but less risky, expected output. On the other hand, the manager of a school district whose residents were less averse to risk might choose the newer and more uncertain program.

In sum, the manager's choices in an uncertain world should reflect his constituents' attitudes toward risk. Again, if we redefine the productivity of individual inputs to include their effect on the uncertainty of educational outcomes, we can prescribe the choice of an input combination based on productivity and cost.

EMPIRICAL INVESTIGATIONS OF MANAGERIAL BEHAVIOR

Most of the empirical work on school district managerial behavior performed by economists has involved statistical analysis of district budgets. Such analysis has sought to determine how managers allocate new money among budget categories: classroom teacher salaries, numbers of classroom teachers, other personnel, supplies, maintenance, and so forth. Those who have undertaken this type of analysis generally went on to assume that future behavior with respect to the allocation of discretionary funds would be similar to past behavior. Finally, they used estimated empirical relationships (regression equations) to predict budgetary behavior.

Another line of empirical investigation has attempted to build on the admittedly weak basis of estimates of educational production functions. A substantial body of economic literature reports the results of regressions in which the dependent variable is some measure of the output of education and the independent variables are measures of the quantity of various educational inputs.[2] If the coefficients estimated by such a procedure could be taken as indicators of the relative productivity of different educational inputs, we then would be able to add empirical substance to the normative results discussed in the previous section. In other words, one of the objectives of this line of investigation is to reduce some of the uncertainty with respect to production relationships experienced by school district managers.

Unfortunately, most of the empirical models of educational production reported in the literature have been based on the overly simplified model in which production technologies are known with certainty, the managers' objective is to produce as much of a single output as possible, and all inputs are perfectly elastically supplied. As we have seen, it is a relatively simple exercise to relax these assumptions and modify our normative conclusions appropriately. However, developing empirical estimates based on the more complex model is a much more difficult undertaking, so difficult, in fact, that the literature is only beginning to tackle the problem.

SUMMARY

Economic models of school district internal decisionmaking are not as well developed as other aspects of school finance analysis. Theoretical models are largely normative. They suggest that an efficient school district manager will choose combinations of inputs to purchase by comparing the prices of those inputs with their productivity. The productivity of any given input is considered within the context of its role as one of a combination of inputs. Productivity also is defined broadly to account for the relationship between any one input and all of the outputs the district may produce. Factors such as uncertainty about productivity relationships may also be incorporated into the model.

Empirical models of managerial behavior have been ad hoc, producing estimates of the proportions of new money that will be devoted to various budgetary categories.

2. Three of the more recent and insightful of these studies are Brown and Saks (1975, 1980); Summers and Wolfe (1977).

II THE ECONOMIC ANALYSIS OF SCHOOL FINANCE REFORM

7 OBJECTIVES, CONSTRAINTS, AND INSTRUMENTS

This chapter begins with a discussion of two broad topics: the conceptual framework for the economic analysis of a policy issue and the values underlying the call for school finance reform. The conceptual basis of our discussion, "constrained maximization," provides a formal structure for our thinking about reform. Once the structure has been outlined, we proceed to define the objectives, instruments, and constraints associated with school finance reform so as to fit into this framework.

The second section, a discussion of school finance values, formalizes our thinking about the objectives of reform. The section identifies three distinct values that might, to varying degrees, express the preferences of participants in the process of reforming policy. The section also discusses the educational voucher system, the rejection of which may reflect a specific value orientation that should be accounted for in an analysis of school finance. Subsequent sections treat the institutional, macroeconomic, and sociopolitical constraints on school finance reform and the instruments of reform, namely, regulations and grants.

THE CONSTRAINED MAXIMIZATION FRAMEWORK

Recent school finance reform activity has many objectives, not all of which are subject to economic analysis. Some reformers may view the process of changing school finance institutions as an opportunity to organize political coalitions so as to influence legislation only peripherally related to educational issues. Others may value education as an end in itself or have a financial interest in the schooling industry and see finance reform as a lever with which to pry more resources from a reluctant legislature. Some of the goals of school finance reform are, however, subject to useful economic analysis.

Most school finance reformers consider the current distribution of educational resources to be suboptimal and believe that social welfare could be improved by a different allocation of educational services. School finance technicians have proposed a number of policy changes intended to improve this allocation. This and subsequent chapters demonstrate how the techniques of economic analysis can be used as tools of policy analysis to evaluate alternative approaches to reform.

To apply the techniques of economic analysis to the specific problem of school finance reform, we must organize our thinking in a specific formal way. Economists are most comfortable with the conceptual framework of constrained maximization. Any constrained maximization problem contains three elements:

1. Objectives
2. Constraints
3. Instruments

The objectives involved in any policy analysis derive from social values. In fact, the typical objective of policy is to maximize social welfare. Of course, social welfare is a subjective criterion and may subsume a wide variety of specific value judgments. The objectives may include a more even distribution of well-being among households, or they may include only aggregate well-being without regard to its distribution. We may value for its own sake the quantity of some specific output—clean air, for example—produced by the economy. The constrained maximization framework requires only that the social values to be achieved be stated explicitly and subject, in principle at least, to quantification.

This requirement severely limits the generality of the constrained maximization approach. Political maneuvering frequently requires that participants conceal their values. Some social values, such as patriotism or the beauty of public buildings, are not quantifiable.

Economists concerned with the analysis of school finance believe that the values involved in this area are sufficiently quantifiable and subject to sufficient candor to allow for useful economic analysis.

If we always were free to reach all of our social objectives, we would be living in utopia. We are not. We are constrained in the degree to which social values can be realized. The scarcity of factors of production prevents us from making everyone as happy as he might be. The constitutional constraints that we place on government activities prevent our allocating or reallocating goods as freely as any individual might like, given his subjective social values. Hence, the second element of the constrained maximization problem is a precise description of all the physical, social, and institutional constraints that we face in the pursuit of our objectives.

A government has only a limited number of instruments it can use in pursuit of social welfare: It can set tax rates, distribute revenues, and, within limits, regulate the behavior of households, firms, and other institutions. A precise description of these instruments constitutes the final element of the general constrained maximization problem.

The three elements work together in a simple way. The problem is to choose the policy instruments (tax rates, regulations, etc.) so as to come as close as possible to the objectives, subject to the constraints. Of course no one ever has solved an actual school finance problem using the formal constrained maximization approach. The social values, the constraints, and the instruments are all much too complex to allow a straightforward solution. Instead, as with all conceptual frameworks in social science, this approach organizes our thinking and points out potential conflicts or complementarities. An analysis of school finance within this framework may point out conflicts among values, ways in which certain instruments work with and others work against certain constraints, and so on.

THE SOCIAL WELFARE OBJECTIVES OF REFORM

To set up the general school finance problem within the constrained maximization framework, we begin with a discussion of the social values inherent in the objectives of school finance reform.

Identifying School Finance Values

One of our objectives in redesigning, or reforming, a school finance system is efficiency. We have seen that to the extent that education is a public good, the efficient quantity of education will not be provided by a decentralized market mechanism. The pursuit of efficiency, therefore, might dictate a reallocation of resources toward or away from the education sector or a redistribution of resources within the sector. We also wish to raise government revenues, including revenues for education, in ways that minimize dead-weight loss.

There are many ways to improve school finance efficiency and many reasons for doing so. Efficiency might be improved by changing the ways in which governments raise revenue for education. Economic efficiency might be improved by increasing everyone's level of schooling or by decreasing property tax differentials across localities. A case might be made that by improving education for specific classes of children society would benefit more, in terms of increased production, than the cost of the improvement in schooling. Such arguments, however, generally are not made in calls for school finance reform. Most calls for school finance reform are directed at the inequity of the current school finance system, but what constitutes "equity" of a school finance system?

The concept of equity most amenable to economic analysis is distributional equity of income. A highly unequal income distribution is less equitable from many people's point of view than a more equal one. Economists are most comfortable discussing policies involving direct income redistribution, that is, taxing people with high incomes and making money payments to people with low incomes. The attractiveness of a policy of direct income redistribution reflects a specific value judgment, however, and one that is not universally held.

Household Well-Being.   The social welfare function most frequently analyzed by economists values only the subjective well-being of households. Improvements in the well-being of some households may be valued more highly than improvements in other households, but each individual household is assumed to be the best judge of what is necessary to raise its own level of utility.

The government may improve a household's well-being in three ways: by giving it money, by subsidizing its consumption of some good, or by giving it a quantity of some good. If we adopt a policy of in-kind transfers or consumption subsidies, it is only by chance that we will give people exactly what they would have purchased had we distributed the money spent on the program directly. From their subjective points of view, therefore, the recipients will be worse off than they would have been under a program of direct income payments with exactly the same total budget as the in-kind transfer or subsidy program.

Clearly, this traditional framework must be modified if we are to use it to analyze school finance reform. A redistribution of educational services is not an optimal policy if it does no more than improve the subjective well-being of certain groups of households. Recipients of the improved educational services almost certainly would prefer to receive the money directly. Those who advocate school finance reform, therefore, must have some other social values in mind than distributional equity of incomes. Of course, the political strategy of those who value more direct redistribution of income may include the support of school finance reform, but economic analysis cannot deal with the possibility of concealed values.

What values underlie the call for a redistribution of educational services? Why should we be concerned with the distribution of education while we are unconcerned with the distribution of other important goods, such as automobiles and newspapers? Several different value orientations might dictate such concern.

Many of the redistributional policies of federal and state governments in the United States involve in-kind transfers or consumption subsidies of basic necessities. The government provides a food stamp program; before that was instituted, the government directly distributed surplus food to needy households. Public housing programs and Medicaid also involve in-kind transfers or subsidies. The plethora of such programs may reflect the political strength of the agricultural, construction, and medical lobbies, but it may also reflect an aspect of the social values that govern political decisionmaking. It is certainly reasonable to value equitable distributions of certain commodities and services, regardless of how the recipients would have spent the money had they received it directly. Those who oppose this value orientation, however, term the in-kind transfer approach paternalistic.

Our analysis of school finance policy would be incomplete if we failed to consider the possibility that educational services may fall into the category of "basic necessities," but adopting the basic necessities approach does not get us very far in our discussion of the values underlying calls for school finance reform. The objective of the food stamp program is to provide the basic necessities so as to avoid malnutrition. Public housing programs provide minimal shelter by contemporary U.S. standards. School finance reformers, however, aim at insuring everyone much more than a minimal level of educational services. Their objectives may be better described as raising all children's education to the quality now received only by the most privileged. We must, therefore, search further to identify the values behind the dissatisfaction with the current allocation.

Equality of Expenditure.   We begin with the basic justification for governmental involvement in the education sector. Presumably the public good aspect of education is important enough to justify a substantial governmental role in the allocation of this service. At the same time, we require, through such constitutional provisions as the Fourteenth Amendment, that governments provide equal protection of the laws in all of their activities. The equal protection clause, intended to protect minorities from arbitrary action by the majority, can be interpreted as requiring that the allocation of governmental services reflect the application of some legitimate social welfare criterion.[1] In other words, our concern with the allocation of education grows out of the interactions of two distinct values: that the government involve itself in the provision of public goods so as to enhance economic efficiency and that the distribution of any good with which the government involves itself be equitable. The second of these is not an end in itself but, rather, an instrumental value arising out of our desire to protect minorities.

This approach to the social values inherent in calls for school finance reform is subject to somewhat further refinement. Once the government has decided to involve itself in the provision of some service, the service provided to each qualified recipient is presupposed to be of equal quality. Any inequality in the service provided

1. This is not a legal interpretation of the equal protection clause. Courts generally limit their strict scrutiny of the social welfare justification for unequal allocations to cases involving "fundamental rights" or "suspect classifications." These issues would be of central concern were we investigating school finance litigation. At this point, we are saying only that the government's involvement in the provision of education is reason enough to be concerned with the equitable allocation of this good.

should be justified as a means to some social welfare end. This refinement further justifies our scrutiny of the relationships between the allocation of educational services, especially the inequalities in this allocation, and the social values that dictate that allocation.

Preserving School District Integrity.   Most school finance reform activity aims at changes in the distribution of resources among school districts, not among children. For this reason, many of those involved in discussion of school finance reform question the advisability of distributing resources through school districts. They propose instead a system of educational vouchers (Coons and Sugarman 1978; Friedman 1962).

The justification for a voucher system arises fairly directly from a combination of economic theory and a particular set of social values. Suppose we accept the justification for a substantial government involvement in allocating education and also value an equitable distribution of resources among children. At the same time, suppose we value the efficiency associated with market allocations of goods and services. Profit-maximizing firms have an incentive to minimize costs by using inputs in the most efficient manner. Consumers, faced with a wide variety of potential suppliers, have an incentive to take their business to the firm that provides the best services at the lowest cost.

According to proponents of the educational voucher system, by granting school districts near monopoly power over the provision of education within a jurisdiction and by disassociating the supply of schooling from pecuniary incentives, we are denying ourselves some of the efficiency benefits of a market mechanism. After all, the government need not produce a service simply because it pays for that service. Take, for example, the food stamp program: The government pays for food for needy people, but it does not produce or sell that food.

Many school finance activists may accept those arguments but also may have made the political judgment that reform can be achieved more rapidly if it is divorced from the controversial issue of vouchers. They might prefer to distribute educational resources directly to children's parents, but they have decided to accept for the time being an approximation as close as possible to the optimal distribution among children, given that the government subsidizes school districts, not families.

Other advocates of school finance reform may reject voucher proposals not on the basis of political strategy but because a decentralized
supply of schooling would be inconsistent with their values. The
analysis of alternative reform policies will differ depending on
whether the rejection of vouchers is a political expedient or a value-
based choice.

Two value orientations might lead to the rejection of vouchers as an
educational institution. The first relates to one of the justifications for
government involvement in education. Recall that the cohesiveness of
a society depends on shared values and experiences. A fairly uniform
program of public education contributes to the inculcation of these
shared values. If we value cohesiveness, therefore, and judge that the
alternative institutions that would disseminate these values and experiences would not be up to the task, we would opt for governmental
production of education, despite the efficiency cost associated with
centralized production. The charge that a voucher system would
result in many perfectly segregated school systems, one for each
income class and value orientation, reflects the belief that we lack
alternative mechanisms for promoting social cohesion.

The second value orientation leading to the rejection of vouchers as
an educational institution relates to the justification of school districts
as institutions. School districts may indeed be anachronistic. Nevertheless, local education authorities are a lively element of our federal
system and, as such, may be worth preserving. This justification for
school districts as an institution derives from the ideological foundation of our governmental system as best expressed in *The Federalist
Papers.*[2]

Although the most effective way to pursue a public purpose on any
given occasion may seem to be through centralized governmental
activity, we recognize at the same time that too great a concentration
of power in any single agency threatens our liberty. The recognition of
a centralized government's potential for abuse of its authority has
resulted in the balance of powers on the federal level and the division
of governmental powers among several layers of sovereignty. The
preservation of the integrity of each level of government helps to
insure that no single agency becomes too powerful.

2. See especially No. 17. Alexander Hamilton's arguments concerning the protection of
local interests make as much sense with regard to relations between state and local governments
as between federal and state governments.

Thus, while a system of school districts may not be the most efficient mechanism for insuring an optimal distribution of educational resources among children, the preservation of viable local governmental agencies enhances another value, the balance of powers. The voucher advocate's ideal, a federal government distributing "education stamps" to families, might destabilize this balance of powers by short-circuiting state or local governments.

Measuring School Finance Values

The preceding section identified three distinct sets of values that generate a concern for equity in the allocation of educational resources. The first set of values, as always in welfare economics, concerns the subjective well-being of households. In general, our concern for household utility will differ depending on how well the family would fare without governmental intervention. The poor, the handicapped, and those with other economic disabilities may be the subject of special social welfare concern. We may value improvements in well-being more for these groups than for others. In other words, our social welfare function reflects the value of economic efficiency, improvements in everyone's well-being, and distributional equity of incomes. Of course, individuals may differ in the relative degrees to which they value efficiency and equity and in the relative values they assign to improvements in the well-being of any given type of household.

The second set of values involves the distribution of educational resources among children. The values reflected in the equal protection clause require that differences in the resources devoted to the education of different children be justified as means to some identifiable social welfare objective. Disparities must generate a sufficient social welfare benefit to justify the decrease in equality. Therefore, we can translate our equal protection clause into a positive social value assigned to reductions in disparities in the distribution of resources among children.

The third social welfare concern relates to the viability of local governmental institutions. This value is much more difficult than the others to quantify. We measure subjective well-being by assuming that increases in income improve well-being and have a number of ways of measuring disparities in the distribution of educational resources, but the institutional integrity of local governments is a much less rigorously defined concept. We will have to satisfy ourselves with an ad hoc specification of this value.

The independence of a local governmental institution is directly associated with its budgetary discretion. At one extreme is a jurisdiction with independent taxing power and complete freedom to allocate its tax revenues unconstrained by higher levels of government; this might be considered the most viable local institution. At the other extreme is a regional office that may forward information or distribute checks but has no discretionary authority over either the level or the composition of its activities. The middle range of jurisdictional integrity contains local governments that have limited taxing authority and are free to allocate part, but not all, of their budgets as they wish.

What is proposed, therefore, is a two-dimensional measure of local government viability: the proportion of the total local budget allocated at the discretion of local authorities and some measure of the freedom of the locality to levy local taxes. Increases in either of these measures are considered social goods in that they may be expected to increase the integrity of local agencies and, therefore, to help guard against the excessive centralization of power. These are only imperfect indexes of jurisdictional viability. We have no way of measuring the security of local agencies in their authorities. State governments, for example, are protected by the federal constitution and could not be abolished without their own consent. Local governments, while they may have a great deal of fiscal autonomy, are still merely the creations of state governments that in some cases can alter jurisdictional boundaries or limit local government powers at will. This distinction is important but difficult to specify precisely.

The relative importance assigned to these three sets of values—household utility, resource equality, and school district integrity—depends on individual judgment. Some people may not value one or another of these at all. For example, an advocate of vouchers would assign little importance to school district integrity. A strict adherent of the Tiebout hypothesis (1956), valuing school district integrity and economic efficiency, would place little value on expenditure equality. Some school finance litigants, perhaps to stake out a clear adversarial position, seem to value only equality. Our purpose here is not to judge these values but to show how any given set of school finance instruments tends to advance one or another set of objectives.

These values may or may not conflict. Changes in the direction of resource equality may target resources at economically deprived groups. The opposite may also be true. Resource equalization may, on the average, increase or decrease the degree of discretion available to local school budgetary authorities. In other words, the design of an optimal school finance system may involve trade-offs among competing objectives. The final judgment as to which system is best will depend on the relative importance decisionmakers assign to each of the values in the design problem.

THE CONSTRAINTS ON REFORM

The school finance reforms currently contemplated can accomplish only the limited objectives of a redistribution of educational services, a small increase in the average quality of education, and perhaps a small decrease in economic inequality. School finance reform will not in any important way change the major political and economic institutions of our society. Reformers must, therefore, take these institutions as given and treat their structures as constraints on the design of new school finance systems.

In addition, no one expects school finance reform will induce major changes in the pattern of economic development or cultural evolution in the United States. A period of relatively slow, resource-constrained economic growth and of emphasis on increased investments in physical rather than human capital also must be taken as given by reformers, as must the possibility of decreasing public support for government programs in general. The more precise our understanding of these constraints is, the more effective our analysis of alternative policies will be.

Institutional Constraints

Two social institutions dominate the allocation of educational resources in the United States: the system of school governance and the family.

School districts decide on the aggregate level of educational services to provide within their jurisdiction and—what is perhaps more important—determine the allocation of resources among educational programs. The process by which school districts make these crucial decisions involves formal political interactions (elections, school board meetings, etc.), informal political interactions (lobbying, agenda setting, etc.), and bureaucratic procedures.

Each district's allocative decisions are constrained by other institutions (state, federal, and local governments, teachers unions, markets for educational inputs, etc.) and by the resources made available to the district by its own economic environment. Other elements of the school governance system—state authorities, the Department of Education, school principals, teachers, and so on—also play a powerful role in allocating educational resources.

Families also play an important role in determining what kind of education, and how much of everything else, their children get. Families choose where to live, whether to send their children to public or private schools, and what nonformal educational experiences their children will have. They participate, to differing degrees, in the political processes that lead to school district allocative decisions.

All of the choices that families make are constrained. Decisions about private schooling and residential location are constrained by the family's income. Locational choices may also be constrained by zoning or racial discrimination and certainly will be influenced by considerations other than the quality of local schools—by job location, for example. Within these constraints, however, our economic system allows families complete latitude.

A number of factors relating to the institutions that influence educational allocations—the workings of the system of governance, the free economic choices of households, and patterns of residential zoning and racial discrimination—are, then, largely beyond the control of school finance reformers or legislatures. These factors are therefore ignored in any analysis only at some risk. For example, the intent of a reform proposal requiring a substantial reduction of services in high-spending districts could be thwarted by a flight to private schools. A low-spending district's budgetary windfall might have no effect at all on the services provided by the district if the local supply of educational resources were inelastic, or a windfall might exacerbate intradistrict inequalities if the political structure of the district so dictated.

Macroeconomic and Sociopolitical Constraints

A simple projection of recent macroeconomic and sociopolitical trends in the United States does not bode well for the educational sector, especially for essentially redistributive programs within that sector. The attention of high-level policymakers is and will be absorbed by international issues, as well as by such national macroeconomic variables as the rates of inflation and personal savings and the transition from fossil-fuel-based technologies to renewable energy sources.

Household saving is the source of newly created capital, that is, new investment. Investment can take two forms: investment in physical capital, namely, buildings, machines, rail lines, and so on, and investment in human capital,[3] namely, improvements in the health or skill level of the work force.

While the solution of the most widely publicized economic problems—inflation and the energy crisis—undoubtedly will require a great deal of skill and many new ideas, arguably our more pressing need is for more and different physical capital. We need a more energy-efficient and productive aggregate manufacturing plant. We need a new and more fuel-efficient aggregate stock of automobiles and new public transportation networks. A large proportion of our housing stock must be modified with energy conservation in mind.

All of these transformations are taking place, and they will absorb a large fraction of available investment funds for several years to come. The next decade, therefore, is unlikely to witness substantial increases in aggregate investment in human capital—in funding for education.

Several sociopolitical trends are also working against increased investment in education. First, the decline of the birthrate has led to the decline of public school enrollments. The decrease in the school age cohort has two components: a continuation of the slow decline in the number of children per family and, more important, a decrease over the past twenty years in the proportion of potential parents who actually have children. We might expect that a decrease in family size would lead to an increase in the quality of education each child receives. However, the dominant cause of recent enrollment declines

3. One who forgoes the income he might receive from a job so as to attend school or a training program is, in effect, saving. Any saving involves forgoing current consumption to increase future consumption.

works in just the opposite direction. The political process leading to the choice of the "official" social welfare function involves an aggregation of individual value orientations. As fewer adults have children, a decreasing proportion of the population places a high relative value on education. We can expect, therefore, that as enrollments decline the values that inform allocative policy decisions will shift away from support for public school services.

Second, public support for most governmental activity is declining (Pascal et al. 1979). The passage of Proposition 13 in California and of similar measures in other states are aspects of a fiscal limitation movement. This trend suggests that funds available for redistributive programs are unlikely to increase in the future as rapidly as they have in the past.

Finally, the proportion of households choosing private schooling for their children is increasing. While total private school enrollment may decline along with public school enrollment, the desegregation of public schools and the general increase in household real disposable income result in a higher proportion of children in private schools. This trend also leads to diminishing support for expenditure on public education.

To be sure, some sociopolitical trends are working in favor of public school spending. Court and legislative mandates requiring new educational services for previously poorly served groups create a demand for a reallocation of school resources, and the increased political power of teachers' unions may insure that these new requirements are met with new spending and not merely by a reallocation of existing resources.[4]

How can these complex and conflicting trends be reduced to a precisely specific constraint on the design of school finance policies? The simplest way to recognize the resultant effect of these constraints is to place some limit on the total resources available to be spent on educational services. Just exactly what the dollar value of that limit is likely to be at any time in the future is, of course, unknown. However,

---

4. The rise in power of teachers' unions might work in the opposite direction as well. By raising the cost of teachers' services to school districts, unionization may make education of any given quality more expensive. Voters or school district managers may, therefore, be induced to "buy" less education than they might have otherwise. In the long run, though, higher teacher salaries might attract higher quality teachers to the profession. The net effect of these tendencies on the aggregate quantity and quality of education depends on a number of parameters of the labor market for teachers. A discussion of this market lies beyond the scope of this study.

the combination of trends we have discussed suggests that the proportion of total gross national product (GNP) devoted to public elementary and secondary education will not increase over the next decade; in fact, it is likely to decrease somewhat.

We have identified three sets of constraints that limit our options in choosing a school finance system: (1) processes of decisionmaking by school districts and other governance institutions; (2) decisions of households as to where to live, whether to attend public schools, and how to vote, along with the constraints on those household choices; and (3) a fixed or declining proportion of GNP to be spent on public educational services.

THE INSTRUMENTS OF REFORM

The two broad categories of instruments of central (state or federal) government education policy enter into discussion of school finance policy: regulation and intergovernmental grants.[5]

Regulation

The explosion in the number and scope of state and federal regulations of school district behavior over the past twenty-five years is well documented (Wise 1979). Before the 1954 Supreme Court decision, *Brown v. Board of Education,* almost no federal rules regulated district behavior. State regulations were confined, for the most part, to limiting local tax rates requiring the provision of certain curricula or establishing certification requirements for teachers. Since then courts, legislatures, and central educational authorities have expanded the scope of regulation to include many aspects of intradistrict allocation of funds, provision of specialized services to certain categories of students, adoption of specific evaluative procedures, assignment of students and teachers to schools, choice of materials and designs in the construction of school buildings, and so on. Some of these regulations accompany funds distributed through intergovernmental grants or are

5. The provision of a complete technical guide to school finance systems is not among the purposes of this study. The Education Commission of the States' *School Finance Reform: The Wherewithals* (1975) and other publications provide thorough source material on how to design new school finance laws.

conditions for qualification as a recipient. Other regulations are not tied to any state or federal funds.

To analyze the regulation of school district behavior, we can apply a methodology similar to that devised by economists specializing in the field of industrial organization to analyze the effects of governmental regulation on the behavior of firms. Firms may be expected to alter their behavior so as to reduce the burden placed on them by regulation, just as they alter their behavior in response to the burden of taxes. One possible response is, of course, to comply strictly with the regulation, leaving all other decisions—level of output, choice of inputs, price of output, and so forth—as they were before the regulation was imposed. More typically, a firm may be expected to alter some behaviors apparently unrelated to the regulation. A rule limiting the amount of air pollution a firm is permitted to generate may result in a reduction of emissions, but it also may induce firms to reduce output or use different inputs. These changes in behavior will produce economic costs and benefits that must then be evaluated according to some set of social values.

Analyzing the effect of educational regulations is, however, a more delicate task than analyzing the effect of industrial regulations. The simplifying assumptions with respect to the objectives of regulated institutions—namely, profit maximization and cost minimization, which appear to work fairly well in modeling responses of firms—are much less useful as paradigms of school district behavior. Still, the methodology of associating alternative responses with specific objectives of the regulated institutions applies as well to districts as to firms.

The social welfare consequence of a regulation will differ, depending on districts' behavioral responses. One district required to provide a new educational program for, say, handicapped students may respond by raising local taxes, complying with the regulation, and leaving all other educational programs as they were. Another district may meet the new requirement by shifting resources away from programs that are not mandated by central regulation, leaving local taxes unchanged.

Likewise, the social welfare consequence of a revenue limitation will differ, depending on districts' responses. Some states have attempted to reduce disparities in the quality of education among districts by limiting strictly the rate at which already high-spending districts may increase their budgets from year to year. The welfare evaluation of this policy instrument depends crucially on whether the residents of high-spending districts accept this limitation and continue to send their children to the public schools. They may, instead, attempt to maintain the relative quality of the education their children receive by sending them to private schools.

Grants

In designing a school finance grant policy, a government must consider four major programmatic elements: recipients, sources of funds, aggregate levels of funding, and allocation formulas. It first must identify the recipients of the grant: school districts, multidistrict authorities, schools or other subdistrict units, or households.

Second, the central government must decide on the source of funds for the school finance program. For a state government, the source of funds must be current-year taxes, and the choice of tax instruments will influence the social welfare effects of any reform. The federal government has the additional option of increasing the total public debt, and this alternative also will have different social welfare consequences from an increase in one or more of the federal tax rates.

Third, the government must determine the aggregate level of funding of a school finance policy. The choice of a funding level and the design of a formula should not be viewed as entirely separable decisions. Some formulas may work better at high levels of funding than at low levels. For example, a funding formula that includes a wide variety of individual student characteristics and therefore encourages highly individualized programs may be inappropriate in a state in which aggregate funding is inadequate to provide more than a minimal basic program.

Fourth, the government must devise a formula to determine how much each recipient will receive. In computing this amount of money, the formula design must incorporate two sets of choices: (1) the characteristics of the recipients to be included in the formula and (2) the relative weights assigned to each character that is included. Among the obvious candidate elements for inclusion in the funding formula are the number of pupils in the district, some measure of the fiscal condition of the school district, the characteristics of the pupils, the density of school district population, and the physical condition of the district's capital stock.

Once the elements of the formula have been chosen, the relative weights must be assigned to each of them.[6] How much more money will a district receive for each additional child with some special characteristic—a physical handicap, say—than it would receive for a child with no special characteristics? How much more or less will a district receive given a change in population density than it would receive in response to a change in district fiscal capacity? The technical and policy-analytic literature on school finance is filled with nominations of candidate formula elements, along with arguments justifying one or another set of relative weights.

The choices of formula elements and weights is an interactive process. In the context of a social welfare maximization problem it works as follows. We begin with a prespecified set of values or objectives—a social welfare function. We then choose a set of formula elements and experiment with a variety of different relative weights to determine the outcome, in terms of social welfare, associated with each set of weights. One of these sets of weights will maximize social welfare, given the set of formula elements we began with. Then we choose some other set of formula elements and repeat the process of experimenting with weights. Again, we find the weights that maximize social welfare, given the second set of formula elements. We repeat this process with a variety of combinations of formula elements. Finally, we compare the values of social welfare generated by each separate combination of formula elements, weighted optimally. The elements and weights associated with the highest value of social welfare constitute the optimal formula.

This procedure is similar but not identical to the familiar process among school finance practitioners of running a variety of alternative formulas through a computer that calculates and reports the distribution of grants among districts generated by each formula. Each policymaker then evaluates each reported distribution in light of his subjective value judgments or political perspectives and chooses the "best" formula.

The prescribed optimization procedure has two advantages over the typical computer evaluation. First, the optimization procedure

6. We are not speaking here only of what is usually called pupil weighting. A categorical program also implies some weight for certain kinds of pupils in the formula that determines how much money each district will receive. There are two basic differences between categorical programs and simple pupil weighting. First, pupil weighting schemes need not include regulations about how the extra money associated with certain kinds of children is to be used. Second, categorical programs appear as line items in state budgets and therefore may be subject to closer legislative scrutiny than pupil weights.

requires the "prespecification" of values. Second, and more important, the optimization process involves an analysis of the behavioral response of recipients and households to each proposed formula.

More Specific Grant Instruments

A more detailed description of some of the specific forms of intergovernmental grants will facilitate the discussion of response models in the next two chapters. The economic literature on grants distinguishes among these instruments along two dimensions. The types of grants may be illustrated in the two-by-two matrix in Figure 7–1.

The distinctions among types of grants refer to the elements included in the grant formula. If the formula that determines how much money a district receives includes an element representing the level of revenues generated from the district's own tax base, the district's tax rate, or some other measure of local effort, the policy is termed a "matching grant." The central government matches some proportion of the resources raised from local sources. If the district's own revenue decisions make no difference in the amount of money the district receives, the dispersal mechanism is called a "block grant." These two forms of grants are expected to have different consequences for the behavior of school districts.

Matching grants, in effect, reduce the price district taxpayers must pay for each unit of educational services they buy. Recall that in Chapter 3 we defined a concept called the tax price. This was the amount each resident had to pay if educational expenditures per pupil were to be increased by one dollar. Drawing an analogy between school district choices and consumer decisions, we saw that the lower the tax price, the larger the quantity of educational services the district was expected to buy. A matching grant reduces the tax price. If for

Figure 7–1.   Intergovernmental grants matrix

	Block	Matching
General		
Special		

every dollar of local sources the state pays the district, say, 25 cents in intergovernmental aid (a matching rate of 0.25), then the district need raise only 80 cents in local revenues to realize one dollar of total revenues.[7] Block grants, being invariant with respect to school district choice, have no such consequences.

Another way of comparing block and matching grants is based on the possibility that the entire amount of an increase in the grant received by a school district will not be translated directly into increases in educational spending. Some of the additional revenue is likely to be used to decrease local taxes. These alternative uses of the grant funds are analyzed by envisioning a consumer faced with a choice between two goods—education and "everything else." To the extent that the grant is used to provide tax relief, the funds are used by the residents to purchase more of everything else. Matching grants provide an added incentive, a reduction in the price of education relative to the price of everything else, for greater spending on education. Block grants provide no such added incentive, and, consequently, we expect a matching grant program to induce a greater increase in aggregate educational spending (local funds plus central government grants) than would a block grant program with an identical budget.

The second dimension along which we distinguish grants indicates the degree to which the central government specifies the uses to which the funds may be put. The most "general grant" program administered by the federal government is General Revenue Sharing. The funds that state and local governments receive under this program may be used for almost any purpose, except, in fact, to augment local school budgets directly. The federal government also administers the impact aid program for school districts. Localities receive funds in proportion to the number of children of federal government employees served by the district schools. The uses to which districts might put these funds are fairly unrestricted. Most state aid to local districts, such as uniform grants per pupil and equalization aid, can be used for any general educational purpose.

Most federal school aid and a substantial portion of state aid comes to districts in the form of categorical or "specific grants." Such funds must be spent on a specific educational program (e.g., compensatory

7. If the district raises X cents it will receive $.25X$ from the state and be able to spend $X + .25X = 1.25X$. To be able to spend one dollar, it must raise 80 cents: that is, if $1.25X = \$1.00$, then $X = \$.80$.

education, remedial programs, programs for the handicapped, and vocational education) or on some other specific category of school district activity (e.g., pupil transportation, school lunches, and asbestos removal).

According to the categories of educational policy described earlier in this chapter, specific grants actually consist of a combination of an aid formula element and one or more regulations. The grant formula sends districts money in proportion to the number of their students in the category of special concern to the central government, such as the poor, those who are achieving below grade level, the handicapped, and so on. The regulation requires districts to spend at least as much as they receive under this element of the grant formula on the particular activity under consideration. Occasionally districts are required to spend some of their own resources on the aided activity.

Either of the two components of a categorical program, the formula element or the regulation, may be adopted separately. A central government may distribute general aid in proportion to the number of children in certain categories, or it simply may require certain programs and let districts raise the requisite resources on their own. The question for policy analysis is, Which of these approaches—pure general aid, pure regulation, or categorical aid (i.e., a combination of grants and regulations)—is the best instrument for enhancing social values?

SUMMARY

Any optimization problem consists of three elements: objectives, policy instruments, and constraints. The solution consists of a description of which instrument or combination of instruments is the most effective means to any given set of objectives, given the constraints. The constrained maximization framework for the general school finance problem is summarized in Figure 7–2.

The objectives of school finance reform consist of three social welfare values—household well-being, expenditure equality, and school district integrity—the relative importance of which is a matter of subjective judgment.

We have available a wide variety of instruments, made up of a large number of possible grant formulas and regulations in an equally large number of combinations. We also have a variety of possible objec-

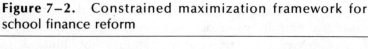

Figure 7–2. Constrained maximization framework for school finance reform

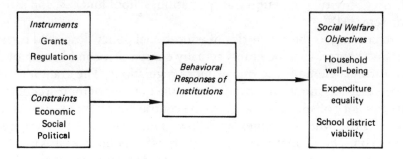

tives, that is, different relative weights assigned to the three main components of social welfare. The goal is to determine which instruments lead to which social welfare outcomes.

To make this connection we need to make an informal guess as to what the behavioral outcomes will be. Which households, if any, will be made better off by the application of any given set of policies? Which, if any, will be worse off? Which policies will enhance expenditure equality and at what cost in terms of other social values? Which policies will best preserve the fiscal integrity of school districts and at what cost?

Economists and others are willing to provide tentative answers to these questions. The answers will be generated by the application of some model of the behavioral responses of school finance institutions—school districts and families—to the opportunities offered or removed by these policy instruments. The consumer of these answers will be better able to evaluate the information provided to the extent that he understands how the conclusions were arrived at.

The next task, therefore, is to examine the behavioral responses of the institutions involved. We do this with a behavioral response model.

8 A COMPLETE RESPONSE MODEL

The reform of a school finance system is a long-term, and therefore risky, undertaking. Because legislative and judicial processes consume a great deal of political energy, major reforms take place only at infrequent intervals. A new basic concept of school finance therefore will remain in place for at least several years, and if the experience of this century is any guide (the recent flurry of legislative activity and litigation notwithstanding), a new system will endure for decades. For this reason, a mistake by a court or legislature is likely to affect adversely the well-being of children and households for a fairly long period.

The risk of error inherent in school finance reform arises because both the school environment and the national economic structure change. A school finance system designed under one set of economic and political conditions may be ill-suited to the circumstances of several decades later. The system designed in the early years of this century by Cubberly, Strayer, Haig, and Mort in an environment of rich cities and poor rural districts cannot easily be adapted to the current environment of poorer cities and wealthier suburbs. Second, major long-range structural changes in the economy are extremely difficult to predict. Three decades ago, for example, few would have predicted the massive suburbanization of whites and northward migration of poor rural blacks. Little can be done, therefore, to reduce the risk that the social environment will outgrow any given school finance system.

A court or legislature's primary objective in ordering or enacting a school finance reform may be to design a system that is desirable for either its procedures or its outcomes. If procedural equity—that is, designing a fair law—is the primary objective, then the analysis may focus on the legislation itself, without regard to outcomes. Such evaluations of procedures fall into the domain of lawyers and political theorists. If, however, the objective is the realization of some set of distributional social values, then the analysis must focus on the outcomes generated by the new school finance system. The outcomes of interest are the well-being of households, the equality of expenditures, and the institutional viability of school districts (see Chapter 7 for a discussion of how these values were identified).

Our knowledge of the outcomes generated by any given change in a school finance system is imperfect, and the design of new systems is therefore risky, but legislatures may be helped in the system design process by a behavioral response model. Economic analysis based on such a model can provide information, admittedly imperfect and incomplete, regarding the most likely outcomes of a given reform. Other behavioral analysis might use models emphasizing the political, social, educational, or psychological aspects of the response to a new school finance system. An economic behavioral response model will emphasize economic determinants: prices, quantities, locational choices, and so on. Because of the imperfections and incompleteness of economic response models, however, unqualified or unexamined acceptance of the predictions of such models may be even more risky than the design of policy in the absence of any information at all.

Response models can be useful in two ways, both of which require an understanding of how the models work and not merely a reading of a computer printout of predictions. The process of building, testing, and critiquing successively more appropriate, inclusive, or refined models of the actions of school finance institutions deepens our understanding of the phenomena under consideration. Model construction and destruction are at least as useful elements of social scientific discourse as the results generated by any given individual model. The types of data related to school finance that have been collected in the past, or could be collected in the future, are both numerous and complex; the potentially telling empirical facts that might be discerned by analysis of such data are equally abundant.

Response models tell us which data would be most useful to collect and which facts most important to know; a complete response model, one that allows for all of the possible outcomes of a change in school finance institutions, will tell us just where any given bit of information fits into a broad map of the school finance world. In other words, a complete response model will tell us not only what we already know or should find out first but also what we do not or cannot know. Both kinds of information are important: the former because knowledge reduces risk, the latter because an understanding of irreducible risks also improves decisionmaking.

The economic literature already contains a great deal of information about the responses of school finance institutions to reform. If, as is likely, interest in these issues continues, much more such information will be produced over the next few years. The purpose of this chapter, therefore, is to present a fairly complete response model that will provide a list of almost everything we might like to know about the responses to school finance systems.

THE ACTORS AND THEIR OBJECTIVES AND CHOICES

The model describes all of the political and economic actors whose decisions interact to determine the allocation of educational resources. The stage on which the actors play their parts may be a state, a metropolitan area, or the nation.

If we wanted to use this model to generate quantitative simulations of the effects of alternative school finance systems, we would use mathematical expression to represent the motives and choices of each actor. The structure of the model and much of its qualitative analysis can be presented discursively, however, and we follow the latter procedure here. The main actors are consumer households, housing and other firms, school districts, local and state governments, the federal government, and educators.

Consumer Households

As in the basic model of production and exchange, each household is characterized by its endowment of factors of production, its tastes, and its demographic composition. The behaviors of households consist of their economic and political choices. They sell their factors of production and receive income, part of which they use to buy consumption goods and part of which they save by buying new factors of production. Consumers also decide whether to vote in local elections; if they choose to do so, they decide for whom or what to vote. Finally, households pay federal, state, and local taxes.

A school finance response model differs from the general model of production and exchange in several respects. First, we are not interested in markets for all goods. Our concern with factor markets is confined to an interest in each household's income level and the market for real estate. Therefore, all of the information regarding the factor endowments of households can be summarized by two characteristics: the household's income and the value and location of the real estate owned by the household.

Nor are we especially interested in all of the consumption and investment decisions made by each household. Instead, we focus on the outcomes of two specific choices: where the household resides within a state or metropolitan area and whether the household's children attend public or private schools.

One final simplification affects the treatment of households in our model. We need not investigate the behavior of each separate household but can be satisfied with an analysis of the behavior of, and effects of reform on, broad categories of households. The categories we choose will depend on our social values and analytical judgments. If some group—for instance, the poor or families with children—are of special social welfare concern, we will want to be able to distinguish the effects of reform on those particular categories. If we judge that the behavior of certain groups—wealthy families with children, for example—will exert a major influence on the outcomes of a reform, we will pay special attention to the choices of that category of households.

Housing Firms

The economic function of housing firms is to transform land and other inputs into housing units of various sizes and styles. At any given time, the state or region is characterized by an existing stock of housing distributed over the area. The price of housing in each locality is determined by the demand for houses at that location and the quantity and quality of the existing housing stock in the locality. Producers of housing respond to these prices and to the prices of land and other inputs required for the production of housing by deciding how much new housing to produce in each locality. New housing will be produced in the largest quantities in localities where the price of the existing stock of housing is highest relative to the cost of producing new housing.

Other Firms

For purposes of school finance analysis, we are more interested in the locational behavior of firms than in their other decisions. Firms pay taxes to school districts; therefore, the decision of a firm to locate in one district rather than another may influence the allocation of educational resources.

As with all of their other decisions, firms choose locations to maximize profits. Locational choices are determined by the differences in the cost of operations in different locations. Firms will be attracted to places that are geographically close to their customers, where the prices of labor, land, and other inputs are low, and where taxes are low. Since school finance institutions influence many of these variables, the locational responses of firms will play a role in determining the eventual outcome of a reform.

School Districts

A state or metropolitan area is assumed to be divided into a number of semiautonomous school districts. At any given time, each district is characterized by an existing physical plant, a set of contracts with current employees, and some general reputation for quality. The latter depends in part, but only in part, on past expenditure behavior.

Like firms and households, school districts make choices. They pursue objectives and are subject to constraints. The choices made by school districts consist of decisions about levels of taxation and expenditure and the assignment of pupils, teachers, and resources to educational programs. As we have seen, though, modeling the objectives of school districts is not as theoretically straightforward as our treatment of the goals of households and firms. Certainly the preferences of the resident households influence the objectives of school districts. The subjective values and goals of district managers possibly influence the decisions independently of the values of residents. To specify our model of district behavior, we must assume some decisionmaking process that will aggregate and reconcile different values. Some variant of the managerial choice model or the median voter model seems the most likely candidate (see Chapter 3).

School districts pursue their objectives subject to constraints. Among these are the regulations on taxation, allocations, and pupil and teacher assignment imposed by state and federal governments. The economic environment of a school district also constrains its choices. Local real estate and other factor markets determine the district's tax base. The location of households influences both the tax base and the demographic composition of the district's population.

Nonschool Local Governments

The state or metropolitan area also is divided into a number of semiautonomous, general local governmental jurisdictions. The choice processes of these institutions are at least as complex and difficult to model as those of school districts, but since the decisions of local governments influence the allocation of educational resources in indirect, but powerful, ways, their behavior must be accounted for in a response model.

Three choices of local governments are relevant: the level of general taxes, the level and distribution of the service budget, and the nature of zoning regulations. Local fiscal and zoning decisions influence the magnitude and composition of the local tax base, which is shared by the school district, and the demographic composition of the local population.

State Governments

The state government is the central policymaker in the field of school finance. Its aid program and regulations are what economists call "control variables" or policy instruments; they are not elements of a response model per se but are, rather, the forces to which other actors respond. However, states do more than aid and regulate education.

They raise general purpose tax revenues to fund a whole variety of programs. Changes in the school finance system may require changes in the level or structure of state taxation or in the budget allocations to other categories of state activity. These behavioral responses of state governments may, in turn, influence the choices of other economic actors who play a more direct role in allocating educational resources.

As sketchy as our understanding of the determinants of local government behavior is, our knowledge of state government behavior is even less developed. Nevertheless, some accounting of the overall adjustments in state policy induced by a change in school finance institutions is an essential part of a complete response model.

The Federal Government

The federal role in the financing and regulation of education has grown markedly over the past fifteen years. If federal aid formulas and regulations were well defined and stable, the federal role could be viewed as a set of available funds and constraints. Federal law, however, allows Department of Education officials some latitude in defining and enforcing many provisions of the law, and many grant programs are competitive or discretionary, rather than formula-driven. Therefore, changes in state school finance institutions and the local response to those changes may elicit different behavioral responses by federal authorities.

As long as we have no predictive theory of federal government behavior, this element of the response model will have to remain ad hoc. Again, our response analysis will be incomplete unless we attempt at least an educated guess as to what the federal government might do in response to the choices of other actors in the model.

Educators

Schoolteachers, administrators, and other education professionals as individuals or as groups make decisions that influence the allocation of educational resources. Potential teachers decide whether to enter the profession and, occasionally, in which district or school to teach. The objectives of individual educators are essentially the same as those of other individuals or households in the model. They sell their labor services for income and purchase consumer goods. They attempt to do as well as they can with what they have. Educators also may pursue specific objectives that are not necessarily shared by other households. Professional norms and peer ratings, along with general consumption, may be important to teachers and principals.

Educators also influence the allocation of resources to and within the education sector through their unions or other professional organizations. Local teacher unions may bargain collectively and strike and thereby influence the expenditure and service outcomes in a school district. State and national teacher organizations may lobby for greater educational expenditures.

The objectives of these organizations are more difficult to model than those of individual educators. The mechanisms by which the values of the membership are combined into a set of organizational objectives are at least as complex as the decision process of a government. As with governments, our understanding of how these organizations operate and how they influence the choices of other actors in the model is poorly understood.

ANALYSIS OF THE MODEL:
INITIAL EQUILIBRIUM

Consider a state or metropolitan area in which a stable school finance system has operated for a fairly long time. In this hypothetical state, as in most states, a large proportion of local school revenues is derived from the property tax. Additional revenues are received through intergovernmental aid from the state and federal governments. Suppose that part of state aid is distributed as a flat grant per pupil and that another part consists of "equalization aid." Districts with relatively low taxable-property value per pupil receive more state aid than wealthier districts. However, the state has made no explicit effort to adjust the school finance formula to insure equal expenditures per pupil among all school districts. Suppose also that the state regulates local taxing authority by limiting property tax levies to a level below some maximum percentage of taxable property value. The federal aid each district receives is determined entirely by the socioeconomic composition of its student body.

The Equilibrium Allocation of Education

Given these circumstances, what will the equilibrium allocation of educational resources among students look like? To answer this question we must define more precisely what we mean by an equilibrium. For the system we have described to be in equilibrium, several conditions must hold. Each household must be maximizing its utility, subject to the constraints imposed by the school finance system and the underlying economic conditions. That is, no household must be in a position to improve its level of well-being either by moving to some other school district or by shifting its children between public and private schools.

At the same time, each school district and each local government must be making choices consistent with the preferences of the households that reside within their jurisdiction. Housing and other firms must be maximizing profits. It must not be the case, therefore, that housing firms could have made greater profits by supplying a housing stock with some other than the observed geographic distribution. The location of different types and qualities of housing is a characteristic of the equilibrium. Likewise, nonhousing firms must be in the locations that maximize their profits.

Now we may describe some of the characteristics of the allocation of educational resources. Obviously, the education each child receives depends on all of the elements of the general equilibrium. The educational resource choices available to each household consist of the expenditure levels of all of the school districts in which that household might choose to live, along with the private schools in the area. These expenditure levels will differ across school districts depending on:

1. The incomes of district residents
2. The tastes of district residents
3. The objectives of school district managers
4. The tax price in the district

The tax price depends on several factors. The cost to each household of an additional dollar of expenditures per pupil—that is, the tax price—will be lower in districts in which the nonresidential portion of the local tax base is relatively large. In other words, the tax price will be lower in places where a large number of nonhousing firms choose to locate. Furthermore, the tax price faced by the average household will be lower if there are a large number of wealthy households in the district. High-income households pay more in property taxes than it costs to educate their children, effectively subsidizing the consumption of education by less well-off local residents. Finally, the tax price is influenced by the rate at which the state matches local revenues. If state aid is not affected by local expenditure choices, then state aid has no effect on tax prices. However, if the state, through its school finance formula, offers to send the district, say, 25 cents for every dollar the district raises from its own resources, the effect is to lower the tax price by 20 percent (see Chapter 3).

The behaviors of firms and wealthy households, which together determine each district's tax price, are influenced in turn by the actual tax and expenditure choices the district makes. Low taxes attract firms and wealthy households. High expenditures attract households with children. The geographic distribution of demand for housing and other consumer goods influences the supply of housing and the location of nonhousing firms across the state or metropolitan area.

What, then, can we expect with regard to the distribution of educational resources? First, it is likely that expenditure levels will differ among school districts. Some districts, especially those that provide good locations for some commercial or industrial activity, will enjoy lower tax prices than others. Districts that offer poor locations for nonresidential activity and do not provide especially desirable residential amenities will suffer high tax prices. Places where low-income people live, usually those districts closest to large central cities, will provide lower-quality education at the lower tax rates their residents can afford.

Second, the residents of any single school district are likely to have relatively homogeneous socioeconomic characteristics. Because the amount of local taxes each household pays is proportional to the value of its house, wealthier households pay more than lower-income households living in the same community. As noted above, high-income households therefore pay more in taxes than the cost of educating their children, while low-income households pay less than the cost of educating their children. When a relatively low-income household with children moves into a community, either the taxes of higher-income households will go up, or expenditures per pupil in local schools will go down. The current residents of the community thus have an incentive to use the zoning power of their local government to exclude new residents with lower income. As a result of such actions, a pattern of income segregation will develop among, communities.

Furthermore, since households choose communities, in part, on the basis of the quality of local schools, those with the strongest preference for education will congregate in the districts with the best schools. For these reasons, then, the equilibrium distribution of households will be characterized by homogeneous groupings of residents in communities.

Finally, it is likely that the fiscal advantages of certain school districts will be reflected in housing values. Districts that are attractive locations for commercial and industrial property or provide residential amenities for high-income households, will, as we have seen, enjoy relatively low tax prices. Such districts will be able to raise relatively high levels of revenues per pupil while levying relatively low tax rates. If the prices of housing were the same in these favored communities as elsewhere, everyone would wish to live there. Such a situation is untenable; therefore, if housing is scarce in the advantaged communities, their residents will have to pay a premium price for housing. This argument can be illustrated quite simply in a supply and demand diagram.

When we say that housing is scarce, we mean that it is somewhat inelastically supplied. Suppose that housing of some given quality is inelastically supplied along identical supply curves in each of two communities. Suppose further that community A enjoys a fiscal advantage over community B, a lower tax price, but that the communities are identical in every other way. At any given price of housing, therefore, more households would prefer to live in A than in B. The demand curve for housing in A lies above the curve for B. These circumstances are illustrated in Figure 8–1.

Curve S represents the identical supply curve in the two communities, D_A is the demand curve for housing in A, and D_B is the demand curve for housing in B. As the figure shows, the equilibrium prices and quantities differ in the two communities. The price of housing is higher in A, and the quantity supplied greater. The larger quantity in A represents the conclusion that under these circumstances the quantity of housing, and therefore the population, of A

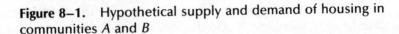

Figure 8–1.   Hypothetical supply and demand of housing in communities *A* and *B*

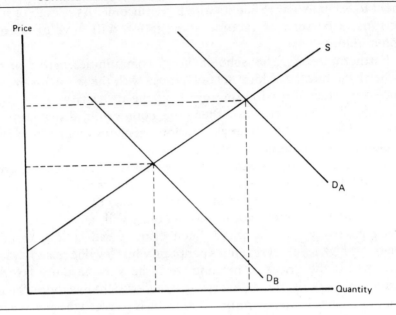

will be greater than that of *B*, even though the two communities are identical in all respects except for their relative fiscal advantages.

The model described by these assumptions is not quite as simple as the circumstances illustrated in Figure 8–1. The complicating fact is that the demands for housing in the two communities are not independent. The higher the price of housing in *B*, say, the higher the demand for housing in *A*, everything else being equal. Figure 8–1 illustrates the equilibrium positions of the two communities once all of these interactions have been taken into account.

What, then, one might ask, determines the relative prices of housing in the two communities in equilibrium? Recall that in equilibrium no household must have an incentive to move. It must be the case, therefore, that all households that might choose to live in either *A* or *B* must be equally well off, regardless of which community they actually live in. Prices and quantities must adjust so that similar residents of the two communities are equally well off. Otherwise the less well-off households would have an incentive to move and to bid up the price of housing in the preferred community.

The conclusion that similar residents of the two communities are equally well off confounds some of the thinking behind school finance reform activities. We frequently observe that while some districts enjoy high spending per pupil and low taxes, other districts suffer high tax rates and low expenditures. Some courts have taken this fact as prima facie evidence of horizontal inequity. However, we see now that similar residents of the two communities may be equally well off. We must look more closely at these two archetypical districts to discern what, if any, inequity exists.

The model on which this conclusion was based is highly simplified. We assumed that residents of a metropolitan area had complete information about tax rates and services in different communities. We assumed that it was not very costly to move from one place to another. In other words, we assumed that there was very little "friction" in the system. A more complex model would allow for such friction and would examine the ways in which imperfect information and a high cost of moving might generate an equilibrium characterized by horizontal inequity. However, the fundamental conclusion of this discussion survives no matter how complex we make our model. The observation of high-spending, low-tax districts along with low-spending, high-tax districts does not constitute prima facie evidence of horizontal taxpayer inequity.

The Effects of a Reform

Suppose now that the state legislature chooses to change the school finance system. More state aid now will be sent to some school districts and, possibly, less to others. Assume, however, that in the average district the state's share of school revenues will increase. To finance this new system, the state will have to increase one of its general tax rates. While the specific outcomes of any given school finance reform will depend on the design of the new aid formula and accompanying regulations, the varieties of possible responses to any reform proposal can be outlined based on a simple analysis of our response model.

The reform will first of all change the pattern of school tax rate and expenditure levels among school districts. Districts receiving more aid will be able to lower taxes, spend more, or both. Districts receiving less state aid will have to raise taxes, lower expenditures, or both.

Since household consumption decisions, including the decision about where to reside, are influenced by a community's school finance characteristics, the reform will induce changes in these consumption patterns. Households that previously might have chosen to live in districts that were relatively well off under the old system may now choose to live elsewhere. Households living in previously low-spending districts while sending their children to private schools may now switch to the public sector. At the same time, though, households that had chosen high-spending districts because of the better-than-average educational opportunities offered may now switch to private schooling. Finally, since some state taxes are increased while some local tax rates are decreased, the distribution of aggregate state and local tax burdens among households will change. As a result, household behavior again will change.

All of these changes will be reflected in the socioeconomic compositions of the student bodies of each district, and the change in socioeconomic composition eventually will change the distribution of federal aid among districts. As the pattern of fiscal advantages and disadvantages among school districts changes, the demands for housing in different locations will shift, and this will induce changes in the price of housing. Houses in previously advantaged districts will experience a drop in relative value; houses in previously disadvantaged districts will rise in value. Accordingly, the owners of these houses will become somewhat wealthier or somewhat poorer as a result of the reform and then will alter their economic behavior in response to their new circumstances.

Firms also may change their behavior. Housing firms now will choose to supply more of their products in the communities that have become relatively more desirable as a result of reform. Changes in the pattern of housing development are therefore likely to follow changes in the demand for housing. Nonhousing firms also may change their locations in response to the new pattern of differential taxation created by the reform and to the new geographic distribution of their customers.

The behavior of general local governments, most notably zoning decisions, is also likely to change as a result of reform. As local reliance on the property tax as a source of revenues declines, the redistribution inherent in the local tax system becomes less important. Recall that under the prereform regime the arrival of a low-income family with children increased the fiscal burden on the wealthier households in the district, creating an incentive for restrictive zoning. This incentive now is reduced because the state is assuming a larger share of the total burden of educational expenditures.

Changes in the economic geography of the state or metropolitan area also will change the size and composition of school district tax bases and therefore will alter the tax prices of school districts. The decision mechanism of the districts will respond to these changes by again altering tax levies and expenditure levels. The other economic actors will respond to these new conditions, thereby inducing further changes, and so on until a new equilibrium is attained.

This hypothetical chronology should be sufficient to illustrate the fact that the response to a school finance reform is of a general equilibrium nature. We are considering several very closely related markets. We expect changes in the allocation of resources in the public education sector and some shifts between the public and private sectors. The outcomes in these two markets influence each other, because the quality of the public sector influences the demand for private education, and political support for public schools is affected adversely by shifts to private schools.

The housing market and the allocation of educational resources affect each other. The education a child receives depends on where his parents choose or are constrained to live. Parental choice and therefore the housing market are influenced by the availability of different qualities of education and different tax rates in different districts.

Finally, the outcome of the change process in any one district is influenced by the outcomes of the process in all other districts. Households choose their residental locations based on the relative quality of schooling and the relative local tax rate in each district. A district's relative desirability depends on how it compares with other districts. The number and type of households and firms that choose to locate in any single district depend on what has happened in other districts. Thus, the outcome of reform in any single place depends on what happens everywhere else.

Once all of the adjustments have taken place, some households will be better off than they were before reform and some will be worse off. The variance in expenditures per child will have changed, and the fiscal independence of school districts will have changed. Therefore, the level of social welfare will have changed. The range of possible outcomes is so wide, given the complexity of the system, that no a priori judgment is possible as to whether any given social values have been enhanced or diminished.

SUMMARY

A complete accounting for all of the possible responses to a change in school finance systems can reduce the risk involved in designing a reform. A number of response models of greater and lesser complexity and inclusiveness have been developed and used by economists involved in school finance analyses. Consumers of school finance analyses will be able to make more thoughtful use of these models if they understand the design and limitations of each particular model and are able to follow, or even join, the process by which ever more sophisticated response models are developed.

This chapter has outlined a complete response model, of which all existing models are simplified special cases. The actors in the model are households, firms, school districts, local and state governments, the federal government, and educators. Our understanding of the objectives and behaviors of these actors varies in depth.

The analysis of this general model points out several characteristics of the behavioral response to school finance systems. First, we see that the allocative choices of school districts and the locational choices of households and firms are closely linked. Second, because the school finance characteristics of any single school district cannot be completely understood in isolation, they should be viewed in the context of the entire distribution of expenditures and taxes in districts throughout the state or metropolitan area. Third, any change in school finance institutions will induce a wide variety of political, economic, and geographical changes, all of which influence our evaluation of the overall performance of the economy.

Changes in the location of residences, the prices of housing, school expenditure, tax rates, and so on will change both the efficiency and equity of economic allocations in directions that are impossible to know a priori. This should be a sobering conclusion for both school finance policymakers and analysts. Policymakers should be concerned because the outcomes of their decisions are not known. Analysts should be concerned because the work that has been done does not begin to approach that which will have to be done if we want to fill in all the blanks in the complete model. Nevertheless, the bits and pieces of work that have been completed have deepened and expanded our general understanding of how school finance systems work.

9 RESPONSE MODELS: THE STATE OF THE ART

The complete response model outlined in the previous chapter may never be constructed or estimated. Every element of the state or metropolitan economy, except for the tastes and before-tax incomes of consumers, the technology of firms, and the geographical boundaries of political jurisdictions, is expected to change as a result of a major school finance reform. Not only may all of the variables change, but everything depends on everything else. Consumer choices depend on the decisions of firms and vice versa. What happens to taxes and expenditures in each district depends on what has happened in every other district. Changes in some of the variables may, in fact, turn out to be very small, and some of the interactions among variables may be extremely tenuous. However, we cannot know a priori which possible outcomes may be safely ignored.

Nevertheless, our understanding of many elements of the ideal response model has become much broader and deeper over the past several years. At the beginning of the 1970s, all we could do was to put a formula into a computer and calculate the resulting state aid distribution, without regard to any change in household, firm, or district behavior induced by reform. By the end of the decade Professor Robert Inman (1978) was able to design, estimate, and use a highly sophisticated response simulation model that allows a great many behavioral variables to change as a result of reform. This chapter concludes with a description of Inman's work. To understand what his model does and does not do, however, we first must understand how each element of his model was developed in the economic literature.

To construct a complete response model we would need to know the relationships between a number of economic variables. Each of these relationships consists of a statement about the effect of one variable on another. Table 9–1 lists most of these relationships, indicating some that have attracted the attention of economists and to what degree of intensity.

Few of the studies discussed below explicitly treat the effects of an actual school finance reform. Instead, the researchers attempt to discern the relationships among the variables by observing the behav-

Table 9–1. What we need to know to build a complete response model

The Effect of	On	Research Reported
State aid formulas	School district spending	Much
School district spending	Differential tax rates	Much
School district taxing and spending	Local property values	Much
School district spending	Locational choices of households	Some
Differential tax rates	Locational choices of households	Some
School district choices	Local government choices	Some
State government taxing and spending	Firm and household choices	
School district spending	Private school enrollment	
Choices of educators	Choices of other actors	
Choices of other actors	Choices of educators	
Changes in each school district	Changes in other school districts	

ior of school districts and households under an established school finance system.

Researchers might, for example, collect data on school expenditures (Y), state aid payments (X), and a number of other school district characteristics (Z, W, V) at some given time and estimate a regression equation of the following form.

$$Y = \alpha_0 + \alpha_1 X + \alpha_2 Z + \alpha_3 W + \alpha_4 V + \cdots \cdot \qquad \text{Eq. (9–1)}$$

If X varies among school districts, as state aid payments usually do, then we can estimate a value of α_1. To use this regression equation to simulate school district responses to changes in the finance formula, we must assume that the behavioral parameters, α_1, α_2, α_3, α_4, and so on will be the same after reform as they were before. If this is so, then we can predict the new value of Y simply by substituting the new value of X. This procedure may generate reliable results, but only if all of the determinants of school district spending have been included in the model and only if none of these other variables, Z, W, and V, change as a result of reform.

As we have asserted and shall show, none of the models developed to date includes all of the relevant variables. Furthermore, as our complete response model indicates, all of the relevant variables could change as a result of reform. This general deficiency could be remedied somewhat if we had data on pre- and postreform behavior of school districts, and such data should become available as more and more states change their school finance systems in significant ways. Analysis of these data would enable us to determine by how much the behavioral parameters do in fact change as a result of reform.

This fundamental conceptual problem also has an econometric aspect. In Chapter 3, we discussed several of the potential econometric problems that might make it difficult to obtain precise and reliable estimates of important parameters. The available school finance data exhibit all of the potential problems discussed in Chapter 3 and a number of others. Each of the studies we discuss in this chapter deals with some of these problems in an appropriate way. Other potential econometric problems are dealt with inappropriately or not at all. A detailed analysis of the econometric procedures used in each study would enable us to evaluate the results in light of the quality of the underlying statistical methodology, but such a digression would detract us from the main purposes of this text. Suffice it to say that many of the uncertainties and inconsistencies in the literature might be resolved by a general improvement in econometric techniques.

STATE AID FORMULAS AND SCHOOL DISTRICT SPENDING

Most of the literature on the effect of state aid on school district spending behavior builds on the work of Bergstrom and Goodman (1973), the pioneers in the empirical application of the median voter model. State aid to the school district is broken down into two segments: a block grant and a matching grant. State aid distributed as a flat-rate grant per pupil or under a foundation plan would constitute a block grant. Guaranteed tax base, percentage equalization, or power equalization would be represented as a matching grant in this context. The value of the block grant enters the regression equation directly as one of the right-hand variables. The matching rate for the school district influences the value of one of the other right-hand variables, the tax price. Other factors that determine the tax price are the nonresidential proportion of the tax base, the median value of housing in the district, the aggregate size of the tax base, the median voter's federal and state tax brackets, and the average daily attendance (ADA) of the district.[1] As the tax price is viewed as the crucial control variable in the model, a deeper understanding of what this variable measures and how it is constructed is essential.

We are after a measure of how much the median voter must pay if expenditures per pupil in the district are to be increased by one dollar. This is the controllable variable that exerts the most influence on behavior in the median voter model. The total tax revenues that must be raised if expenditures per ADA are to be increased by one dollar is simply $\$1.00 \times ADA = \$ADA$. If the state matching rate is m ($\$.25$, $\$.10$, or something like that), then the portion of the incremental expenditure that must be raised from local sources is $1/1 + m$.[2] So $\$ADA(1/1 + m)$ must be raised locally if spending per pupil is to be increased by one dollar. If some proportion, n, of the local tax base

---

1. Since all of the factors that determine the tax price depend on each other and also on the outcomes of the district decision process, the econometric problems involved in isolating the effects of strictly independent variables are quite difficult.

2. We wish to increase spending by one dollar. To do so, we must raise $\$X$ locally, so that $\$1.00 = X + mX$. Therefore, $X = \$1/1 + m$.

consists of nonresidential property, then the residents as a group must pay $ADA(1/1 + m)(1 - n)$. Residents divide their share of the total tax bill in proportion to the value of their houses. The share of the median voter will be Vm/VT, where Vm is the assessed value of the median voter's house and VT is the total assessed value of housing in the district. Therefore, the median voter must pay $ADA(1/1 + m)(1 - n)(Vm/VT)$ more in taxes if per pupil spending is to increase by one dollar. However, the median voter who owns a home can deduct the new property taxes from gross income for purposes of computing federal and state income tax liability. Therefore, the new tax will reduce the median voter's income tax liability by some amount. If the proportion of the local tax increase returned to the voter in the form of a reduction in federal tax liability is f (.5, .25, or something like that), then the actual decrease in after-tax income associated with a one dollar increase in expenditure per ADA will be

$$ADA(1/1 + m)(1 - n)(Vm/VT)(1 - f).^3$$

To specify the tax price faced by the median voter completely, one would have to have data on each of these elements. Not all of the studies reviewed here included all of these factors in their computation of the tax price, and this lack of data may account for some (but not all) of the disparities in their findings.

Among the other independent variables included in the most complete regressions are median income of the district residents, some measure of the distribution of income among district residents, the proportion of dwellings that are owner-occupied, the value of state and federal categorical grants per pupil, and a number of variables intended to represent differences in the "taste" for public education in different school districts. Likely candidates for inclusion in this last category are the proportion of resident children who attend private schools, the proportion of elderly, the proportion of poor, and the proportion of professionals.

The objective of these studies is to estimate response parameters, but, as we have noted, their usefulness for this purpose is uncertain. Our complete response model tells us that two possible outcomes of a major school finance reform will be a rearrangement of households

---

3. This assumes that the median voter is an owner-occupant. If the median voter is a renter, then the formula for the tax price must be modified to include the multiplication factor r, the proportion of tax bills on renter-occupied housing borne by the tenant. If the median voter is a renter, then the tax price will be $ADA(1/1 + m)(1 - n)(Vm/VT)r$.

and firms among school districts and changes in housing values among districts. The relatively simple expenditure-determinant models discussed here allow for only the initial changes in state aid payments to districts. Since all of the other independent variables also might change by an unknown amount, response predictions based on these models are of unknown accuracy.

Nevertheless, these simple models are useful in two ways. First, they may give us fairly good indication of the initial impact of a school finance reform, before some of the behavioral adjustments have worked themselves out. For example, they might be used to predict the outcome of a reform one or two years after reform has taken place—after each district has responded by changing expenditure levels of tax rates but before residents have rearranged themselves among communities or property values have changed. Second, a school district response model is an essential building block of any comprehensive response model. Indeed, we shall see how Inman (1978) used such a model as a component of his simulation procedure.

A summary of the empirical results of some of the studies that have appeared in the literature is presented in Table 9–2. This table leaves out the extensive results reported in doctoral dissertations and in numerous unpublished policy papers. Furthermore, a simple comparison of the numbers in the columns might be very misleading. Each author used different econometric techniques, included different explanatory variables, and worked with different samples of data. Park and Carroll (1979) also reproduced the methodologies previously used by Feldstein (1975) and Ladd (1975); nevertheless, the differences in results between the Michigan and Massachusetts studies remain as they appear in Table 9–2.

On first inspection the results of all of the studies appear reasonable. The price elasticities are negative, indicating, as they should, that the higher the tax price the less expenditure per pupil residents want to buy. Income elasticities are positive, as they should be. The findings also indicate that block grant increases lead to relatively smaller expenditure increases than do matching grant increases.

On closer inspection of the numerical values, however, we note wide disparities, and these are troublesome from a policy analytic point of view. The differences are especially marked between the Feldstein, Ladd, and Inman studies on the one hand and the Park and Carroll work on the other. Since these are the most readily comparable and most sophisticated analyses, we will focus on the differences in the policy implications of these two sets of studies.

Table 9–2. Estimated parameter values in six major expenditure determinant studies
(Dependent variable = Expenditures per pupil)

Study	Sample	Tax Price Elasticity	Income Elasticity	State Block Grant Elasticity
Perkins (1977)	Massachusetts	−1.29	1.07	
Borcherding & Deacon (1972)	Fifty states	−1.23, −1.16	.81, .95[a]	
Feldstein (1975)	Boston SMSA[b]	−1.00	.475	.06
Ladd (1975)	Boston SMSA	−0.485	.495	.03
Inman (1978)	New York City & Long Island	−.41	.60	.37
Park & Carroll (1979)	Michigan	−0.02	.04	.005, .006

[a]The range of estimates represents the results of different specifications of the regression model.
[b]Standard metropolitan statistical area.

Feldstein, Ladd, and Inman found a relatively elastic demand for educational resources with respect to both income and the tax price—meaning, among other things, that even relatively small percentage decreases in the tax price (or increases in income) would be reflected in relatively large increases in expenditures per pupil. If these findings are accurate, then the policies advocated by most school finance reform activists, namely, power or percentage equalization, might indeed reduce expenditure inequalities while retaining school district autonomy in spending decisions. Given the Feldstein, Ladd, and Inman results, the social welfare goals of expenditure equality and school district fiscal integrity do not appear to be irreconcilable.

The Park and Carroll findings indicating a highly inelastic demand do not seem to justify these optimistic policy conclusions. Large changes in the school finance system, according to their findings, would apparently have little effect on expenditure differentials among school districts. As long as local choice is given free reign, expenditure disparities, driven (as they appear to be in the Park and Carroll findings) by taste differences or randomness of behavior, will remain essentially unchanged. Of course, the state could impose any expenditure pattern it liked by assuming all school expenditures. However, this expedient would not resolve the fundamental conflict between the social values of expenditure equality and district fiscal autonomy.

There are two reasonable explanations for the differences between the findings of Park and Carroll and those of Feldstein, Ladd, and Inman. First, for some unidentified reason, voter behavior in Massachusetts and Michigan may differ. This conclusion leaves us somewhat uncomfortable, because an important determinant of behavior is unknown. We can get around this problem, however, by building and estimating different response models for different states. The second explanation is much more troublesome. It may be that some fundamental flaw in the design of these models or in the econometric procedures generates markedly different analyses of essentially similar models.

The resolution of this quandary tops the research agenda of many economists interested in school finance. The first steps should be careful analysis of each study's methodology and, where possible, reestimations of the basic equations in each model, using the best available statistical techniques. Further progress would require more data. A uniform data set for several states, with observations of both individual household and school district behavior over a period of time marked by a major school finance reform, would be ideal for identifying precise parameter estimates.

DISTRICT SPENDING AND TAXING AND LOCAL PROPERTY VALUES

School finance analysts only recently have become aware of the potentially profound implications for their field of a body of literature that has developed over the past dozen years (Gurwitz 1980; Wendling 1979). In 1969, Wallace Oates reported the first of what have come to be called capitalization studies. Oates reasoned as follows: The theory of local public finance is grounded on the assumptions that (1) consumer voters are aware of differences in the quality of public services and levels of local taxation in various communities and (2) they take these differences into account in deciding where to live. If these assumptions are true, according to Oates, then we should expect that consumers would be willing to pay more to live in communities where public services are superior, everything else being held equal, or where tax rates are low, everything else being held equal. If, Oates continued, we could observe the values of similar houses in two communities, identical in all respects (including tax rates) except that one community provided better public services than the other, we should expect to find that the house in the better-served community cost more than the other house. Likewise if two communities were identical in all ways (including the quality of services) but levied different tax rates, we should expect to find that the value of identical houses would differ in the two communities, the value of the house being greater in the jurisdiction with the lower taxes.

This analysis led Oates to estimate the following equation:

$$V_j = \beta_0 + \beta_1 E_j + \beta_2 T_j + \beta_3 X_j + \beta_4 Y_j + \cdots \qquad \text{Eq. (9–2)}$$

In this model, V_j is the median value of houses in school district j. E_j, the expenditures per pupil in j, and T_j, the local property tax rate in j, are the capitalization variables (the concept of capitalization is explained on pp. 81–84). X_j, Y_j, and so on are characteristics of community j (its location in the metropolitan area, the socioeconomic composition of its population, etc.) or characteristics of the housing stock (the median number of rooms, land area, presence of basements, etc.). These latter variables are included to account for the presuppositions in the model that the houses being compared are identical and that the communities are identical, with the sole exceptions of their public finance characteristics.

What would the capitalization coefficients β_1 and β_2 mean in the context of a school finance response model? The most obvious application of these findings would involve the social welfare evaluation of a reform. If reform changes relative property values, some property owners will enjoy an increase in wealth while others will suffer a loss. Since we place a social welfare value on the well-being of each household, the magnitude and distribution of these losses and gains will influence our evaluaton of the reform. Second, recall that the aggregate value of property in each district and the value of each house influence the expenditure choices of districts through their effects on the tax price. If reform changes the values of these variables through the mechanism of capitalization, then precise predictions of expenditure outcomes require some accounting for these induced effects.

Oates, estimating an equation like Eq. (9–2) for a sample of fifty-four bedroom communities in northeastern New Jersey, found that the public finance terms had significant effects in the expected directions. Property values were somewhat higher on average in districts where expenditures per pupil in local public schools were higher, all other determinants of property values being held constant. Property values were higher in communities where taxes were lower, again everything else being held equal.

A large number of studies similar to Oates's original work have been reported in the journal literature and elsewhere (e.g., Edel and Sclar 1974; Brueckner 1979; and Newachek 1979), and the findings have been similar enough to justify some conclusions regarding the capitalization phenomenon. With samples of jurisdictions drawn from within a single large metropolitan area (e.g., Boston, San Francisco, and New York), we generally observe the results Oates expected and found: School finance variables have a significant and quantitatively important effect on property values. With samples of jurisdictions drawn from among regions in a single state or from within smaller metropolitan areas (Syracuse and New Haven), we tend not to observe the expected results.

The contrasting findings of these studies with regard to the effect of school finance variables on property values in large and small metropolitan areas suggest that we might safely exclude property value effects from the design of a school finance simulation model for states without large metropolitan areas. For several reasons, however, this conclusion cannot be considered firm.

First, we do not have a good explanation for the difference in findings between large and small metropolitan areas. The logic of capitalization model makes no reference to the size of the metropolitan area, and we therefore should expect the same findings regardless of the sample analyzed. One ought to be wary of dismissing the importance of a phenomenon on the basis of an essentially anomalous finding.

The second reason for not jumping to conclusions on the basis of even a relatively large set of studies refers to the basic weakness of almost all existing empirical studies of local public finance. Recall that these analyses are based on observations of a stable school finance system. Oates and others are estimating the effects of expenditures and taxes in the average community, given the existing array of tax-expenditure packages in all other communities. If, as a result of a school finance reform, the entire array of tax-expenditure packages were to change markedly, we would expect that the relative attractiveness of the particular expenditure and tax levels in the average community also would change.

It is therefore risky to base firm conclusions about what might happen as a result of reform on simple observations of prereform behavior. Again, this risk can be reduced somewhat by the application of the best econometric techniques to the ideal data. There is room for improvement in the literature on both of these areas.

STUDIES OF OTHER RELATIONSHIPS

Research by economists and other social scientists on other relationships affecting school finance reform is much sparser than analyses of expenditure determinants or capitalization effects. We ought to know more about the effect of school district spending and taxing decisions on household locational choices. Economic theory places great emphasis on this aspect of behavior, and the capitalization studies provide evidence that school finance characteristics to some extent influence housing markets. Capitalization studies alone, however, cannot provide sufficient information about household choice. We know that the average household values high public school expenditures, as evidenced by a willingness to pay more for a house in a district where spending per pupil is high. We do not know which types of households are willing and able to take advantage of high spending per pupil.

We expect, for example, that families with children are attracted to high-spending districts and that childless households prefer places where school taxes are low. Given these incentives, households should sort themselves out among districts. Among households with children, there may be even finer gradations of behavior. Those who value education most highly will be willing to pay the highest premium for housing in high-spending districts. Those with other priorities or opportunities will wind up in places where expenditures are somewhat lower. Merely observing property values without reference to the identity of the households that choose a particular community cannot tell us whether these detailed behaviors take place, much less whether changes in these behaviors are likely to follow a school finance reform.

Econometric analysis of this kind of behavior requires data on the locations and detailed characteristics of individual households and school districts. Such data sets are relatively scarce. Furthermore, it is only in the past decade that the econometric techniques required to analyze such data have been developed. It is not surprising, therefore, that only one such study has been reported in the literature so far.

Ellickson, Fishman, and Morrison (1977) found that jurisdictional characteristics exert a quantitatively small effect on household locational choices. However, he was able to distinguish a strong effect of individual school attendance zones on residential choice. High-income households appear to be willing to pay more than low-income households for locations in elementary school attendance zones with high average incomes.[4] Low-income white households, on the other hand, reveal a relatively strong preference for locations in attendance zones with low proportions of blacks.[5]

Ellickson's findings are interesting but incomplete. Relatively few school or district characteristics have been included in the analysis. However, the findings suggest that if the linkage between school quality and the average income of the attendance zone were broken by a school finance reform, we might observe changes in the locational choices of households.

A second major but largely unexplored element of a complete response model involves the relationships between general local government behavior and school district behavior. One direction of this relationship has received no attention at all. We know almost nothing about how the decisions of school authorities or the structure of the school finance system influence the choices of general government managers. There are a number of possible effects, such as changes in budgets, taxes, or zoning regulations, but no empirical analysis has appeared in the literature.

By contrast, a great deal of polemical and some analytical attention has been paid to the effect of local government choices on school district behavior (Brazer 1974; Netzer 1974; Supreme Court of New York 1974). According to the concept of "municipal overburden," jurisdictions that tax themselves at relatively high rates to finance general government services will have less left over to spend on education (the municipal overburden hypothesis is analyzed in detail in Appendix B). We might therefore expect that high general expenditures or taxes exert a depressing effect on school expenditures. This

---

4. That is, given a house in a high-income attendance zone, the higher a household's income, the higher the price the household is willing to pay for that house.

5. That is, given a house in an attendance zone with a small proportion of blacks, the lower a white household's income, the higher the price the household is willing to pay to buy that house. Those effects remain strong even when the racial or socioeconomic composition of the neighborhood, as distinct from the school attendance zone, is accounted for.

hypothesis has been subjected to some empirical testing, and at least one analyst, Professor Harvey Brazer (1974), has detected a small effect in the expected direction. However, the conceptual underpinnings of the municipal overburden concept have not yet been defined with sufficient rigor to allow for definitive empirical analysis.

THE INMAN MODEL

Inman (1978) took the concept and empirical findings discussed above, added to them in some ways, and combined them into a complex simulation model comprising a behavioral response model and a set of evaluation criteria. This model constitutes the state of the art of economic analysis of school finance.

Inman's simulation of the political economy of metropolitan schools works as follows: School districts respond to one of a number of alternative state policy instruments. Households and firms then alter their behavior. Housing values change, firms alter the geographic pattern of their activities, and families enter or leave the public school system. All of these changes then feed back into the local political decision process, and school districts again alter their spending and taxing behavior. This interaction between school district responses and the behavior of other economic actors continues through several iterations until a new, postreform equilibrium is attained. The new equilibrium is characterized by some allocation of educational resources and some level of after-tax income and income after private school tuition for each household.

Evaluation Criteria

The outcomes of the reform are then evaluated according to each of three systems of social values. The first welfare criterion places no value on the redistribution of well-being among households; the second places a high value on redistribution of utility from the rich to the poor; the third values only equality of educational expenditures. Each alternative policy is fed through the response system, and the effects of each policy are evaluated according to each of the social welfare criteria. The policies are then ranked under each set of social values, as in Table 9–3.

Table 9–3. Evaluation of reform outcomes according to social welfare criteria

	Social Welfare Criteria		
	No Value on	High Value on	Equality of
Policy	Redistribution	Redistribution	Educational
Ranking	of Well-Being	of Well-Being	Expenditures
Best	Policy A	Policy B	Policy D
Second best	Policy D	Policy F	Policy C
•	•	•	•
•	•	•	•
•	•	•	•
Worst	Policy J	Policy D	Policy C

This is as far as any model should go. A legislator simply could inspect these findings and support the policy which best enhances his social values. Indeed, the legislator's job would be just that easy if this model were the final word in response analysis.

Unfortunately, although the Inman model is the most highly developed yet available, it is still far from the ideal model outlined in Chapter 8. Inman's findings are useful guides to policymakers, but their usefulness is circumscribed by the assumptions and lacunae built into the model. Wise use of these results requires a sophisticated understanding of the model's strengths and weaknesses. We will proceed, therefore, to "unpack" Inman's model.

Inman's basic tool is a set of demand curves for expenditures per pupil. Recall that researchers estimated expenditure determinant equations in roughly the following form (Eq. 9–1, p. 147):

$$E = \beta_0 + \beta_1 t + \beta_2 I + \beta_3 Z + \ldots.$$

where E is expenditures per pupil, t is the tax price, I is the income of the median voter, and Z is the value per pupil of block grants received by the district. A number of other variables should be added to the end of the equation, but let us focus now on the effects of t, I, and Z on E.

This equation, with I and Z held constant, is plotted in Figure 9–1. It represents a demand curve for expenditures per pupil. De-

Figure 9–1.   Inman's demand curve for expenditures per pupil E, with voter income and block grants held constant

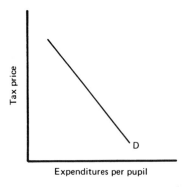

Expenditures per pupil

creases in t will increase the desired level of expenditures. As with the typical demand curve, increases in income will shift the curve to the right, as will increases in block grants. Districts in which the median voter's income is higher or that receive larger block grants will spend more per pupil at any given tax price. These shifts are illustrated in Figure 9–2.

Given one such set of demand curves for each district and a knowledge of the median income, tax price, and level of block grants for each district, we can predict the level of expenditures per pupil in each district. Each school finance reform instrument that might be used by a state legislature will affect one or more of these determinants of expenditures per pupil directly or indirectly. To see how this works, consider a simple reform—an increase in the state aid matching rate to one school district, accompanied by an increase in state income taxes. One set of possible effects of this reform on the affected district is illustrated in Figure 9–3.

Suppose the initial tax price is t_0 and that the increase in the state matching rate reduces this initially to t_1. In the absence of any other changes, we would expect to observe a new higher level of expenditure at E'. The increase in state taxes reduces residents' after-tax income and results in a leftward shift of the demand curve to D'. The outcome then would be a decrease in expenditures from E' to E_1, which is still higher than E_0. Local tax rates might increase or decrease, depending on whether the increased state aid amounted to more or less than the increase in spending.

Figure 9–2. Shifts in demand curve for expenditures per pupil E as a function of changes in income I and block grants Z (Inman model)

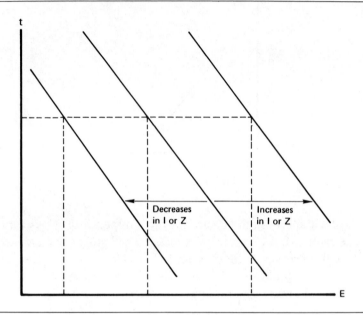

Now suppose that the local tax rate remains unchanged. By assumption, conditions in all other school districts have remained constant. Therefore, this particular district, having been able to increase spending without increasing taxes, is now a relatively more desirable place in which to live. The value of the available housing in the district therefore increases. Because local tax rates did not change, however, the school district is unlikely to have become a more desirable place for firms to do business, and the value of nonresidential property has remained the same. As a result, the nonresidential proportion of the property tax base will drop, and this will raise the tax price facing residents. If this feedback effect eventually raises the tax price to t_2, the final outcome will be E^*, as illustrated in Figure 9–3.

Other, more realistic, state policy options may be similarly analyzed, but they all involve changing tax prices and shifting demand curves in one direction or another for each school district.

Inman also uses his estimated demand curve to predict the number of households that will shift their children into or out of private schools in response to a school finance reform. To see how this works

Figure 9–3. Effects of increase in matching grant rate on expenditures per pupil E (Inman model)

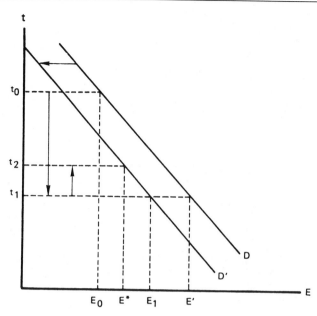

in rough terms, consider a wealthy household in a relatively low-income community. The rich household's demand for education might be represented by D_i in Figure 9–4, the median voter's demand by D_m. At the local tax price, the wealthy family would prefer to consume E_i in expenditure per pupil, but the district offers only E_m. If the wealthy household shifted its children to private schools, its after-tax and after-tuition income would be lower, and its effective demand curve would be represented by D_i'. Even with the lower income, as illustrated in Figure 9–4, the family would still want more education than its local community offered. Such a family therefore very likely would send its children to private schools.

Inman's specification of this part of his model actually involves somewhat greater subtlety than this discussion indicates. However, the simple example serves to illustrate how predictions of postreform spending levels and a knowledge of the income distribution within school districts can be combined to predict how many households will choose the private school option.

Figure 9–4.   Demand curves for high- and median-income households

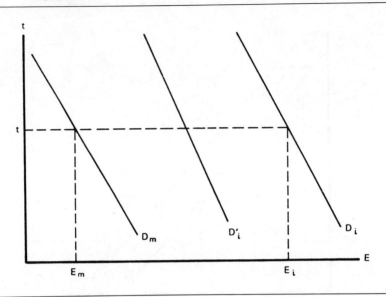

Policies and Results

In the application of his model reported in the literature, Inman simulated the effects of the following six frequently mentioned reform proposals on New York City and fifty-eight suburban Long Island school districts.

1. Foundation aid: A lump-sum payment per pupil to each school district with a tax base per pupil less than some predetermined level. Districts with lower tax bases per pupil receive relatively larger block grants per pupil.
2. Foundation aid with a spending limit: This is the same as foundation aid, but districts are constrained to spend no more than 110 percent of some predetermined expenditure per pupil.
3. District power equalization: This program effectively equalizes the tax bases per pupil of all districts. Identical tax rates among districts result in identical expenditures per pupil. Wealthy districts must return some of their local revenues to the state to be allocated as state aid to poorer districts.

4. District power equalization without recapture: Each district is guaranteed the equivalent of some tax base per pupil. Districts whose actual base is larger than this level receive no aid but need not return revenues to the state.
5. Matching aid: The state pays each district a certain proportion of locally raised revenues. In Inman's particular specification of this plan, the matching rate varies with district mean family income. Low-income districts enjoy higher matching rates.
6. Tax credit: The state grants individual households, as a credit on their state income tax, a proportion of the local school taxes the household pays.

These proposals are compared with each other according to each of the social value systems discussed above, and with the existing state aid plan (a foundation program with a relatively low expenditure guarantee). Increases in aggregate state aid are financed by a proportional income tax. The results of Inman's simulations and social welfare evaluations are listed in Table 9–4.

Table 9–4.   Rankings of policies under Inman's model

	Social Welfare Criteria		
Policy Ranking	No Value on Redistribution of Welfare	High Value on Redistribution of Welfare	Equality of Educational Expenditures
1 (best)	District power equalization	Foundation aid	Foundation aid, spending limit
2	Foundation aid	Tax credit	Matching aid
3	Tax credit	Present system	Foundation aid
4	Present system	Matching aid	Present system
5	District power equalization, no recapture	District power equalization	Tax credit
6	Matching aid	District power equalization, no recapture	District power equalization, no recapture
7 (worst)	Foundation aid, spending limit	Foundation aid, spending limit	District power equalization

Many of these findings are quite surprising. District power equalization (DPE), as advocated by Coons, Clune, and Sugarman (1970) explicitly as an expenditure equalizing instrument and implicitly as a utility redistributing mechanism, turns out neither to equalize nor to redistribute utility very well. Foundation aid, the system that most states have used for the past forty years, turns out to be a desirable policy from the point of view of several different sets of social values, if the foundation level is set fairly highly.

Once Inman explains these results, however, they appear to present a fairly reasonable outcome, given the peculiarities of the New York metropolitan region. Because the vast majority of the region's poor people live in New York City and because that city has a relatively high tax base per pupil, such programs as district power equalization, which equalize tax bases, help the poor very little. Instead they direct state aid to the relatively well-off residents of the (tax-base) poorer suburbs. Because of the capitalization phenomenon, DPE is also a relatively poor equalizer. Initially, DPE lowers tax prices in relatively low-wealth districts, but, as we have seen, once housing markets adjust to the new relative fiscal conditions of school districts, tax prices readjust to close to their prereform levels. The result is a distribution of expenditures similar to what existed before reform took place.

Clearly, Inman's findings cannot be applied directly to other regions. A different distribution of the low-income population, a slightly different set of behavioral parameters, or minor differences in the relative fiscal condition of the central city could easily turn these rankings upside down.

Critique of Inman's Model

Inman has developed and applied one of the most sophisticated tools of policy analysis ever presented in the literature. His subtle synthesis of a wide variety of individual models is clearly a tour de force of economic analysis. Still, like all social science research, his creation is flawed, and for this reason, it can only complement, not substitute for, the factual and value judgments of policymakers.

Some of the inadequacies of the particular application of Inman's procedures are relatively easily remedied within the context of his model in its present design. The policies he described must seem incredibly stylized to anyone familiar with the complexities of the typical state's school finance formula. Density factors, student weighting, categorical programs, and a variety of other appendages to the basic plan could alter radically the ranking of the findings. However, the model easily could accommodate any of these complexities, and the basic framework of simulation and evaluation would work as well for a realistic as for a stylized policy design. Likewise, the welfare orientations according to which policies are evaluated could be made as complex as one might like.

Some fundamental flaws in Inman's system, however, cannot be remedied without a basic redesign of the model or its presentation. First, the only characteristics that distinguish one household from another in this model are family income and residential location. We are unable to distinguish the effects of alternative policies on childless households, on families that place a high or low value on education, and on minority groups.

Second, while Inman allows property values to adjust after a reform, his model does not allow households to move. For example, a household in a previously high-spending district forced to lower its expenditure has only two options: to consume less education or to transfer to private schools. The reasonable alternative of a move to another school district is ruled out. The state of the art of economic analysis, rather than an informed judgment as to the importance of changes in locational choices, forces Inman to limit his model in this way.

Third, like most of the analyses that constitute the components of Inman's model, Inman's analysis depends on observations of behavior before reform to predict behavior after reform. For all the reasons discussed elsewhere, the estimated coefficients in Inman's behavioral equations easily might change as a result of reform.

Finally, the rankings presented as the result of the analysis are not as definite as they appear. The simulation model, and therefore the evaluation of policies, is based on a series of econometric studies. The results of all such studies are characterized by a degree of uncertainty. The data used for purposes of statistical analysis may be faulty. The specification of the econometric model may be mistaken. Some behavior may be random rather than systematic. Because the statistical basis of the analysis is uncertain, so are the simulations and the rankings of the policies. We may be fairly certain that policy B is preferred to policy A under value orientation X but quite unsure that policy C is better than D under Y. The usefulness of these findings would be enhanced if the degree of certainty were known, but estimating the sensitivity of the results of their underlying statistical basis is quite difficult.

Furthermore, we get little idea of how sensitive the rankings are to the specific assumptions made. Suppose that policymakers value educational spending somewhat more than Inman assumes they do. How would the rankings change? Suppose that education is not perfectly elastically supplied. How would the policy conclusions change? The list of such alternative specifications is very long, but the list of alternatives that actually change the rankings might be much shorter. It would be useful to know which assumptions actually affect the rankings.

Policymakers know that households differ along more dimensions than income. Analysts know that people might change their locational choices after reform. Everyone knows that econometric findings have uncertain predictive value. The results of work like Inman's can reduce the inherent risk faced by policymakers, but only if these caveats are kept in mind. Until school finance analysis progresses far beyond Inman's study, there will be no substitute for a policymaker's judgment as to how much the limitations of the model distort the findings.

SUMMARY

Of all of the relationships among relevant variables that might influence the outcome of school finance reform, relatively few have been investigated with any intensity. The two topics about which we know the most are the effect of differences in tax prices on school district expenditure decisions and the effect of differences in taxes and expenditures on property values.

Whether or not state aid formulas can relatively easily reduce expenditure disparities across school districts depends on whether school district expenditure decisions are relatively sensitive or insensitive (elastic or inelastic) with respect to tax price. The econometric problems involved in estimating the tax price elasticity of demand are complex and difficult. Nevertheless, several economists have tackled these problems. Several studies have estimated this elasticity to be in the range of −.41 to −1.00. However, one well-done recent study estimated this crucial elasticity at only −0.02.

Studies of capitalization have found fairly consistently that within large metropolitan areas school finance variables do in fact influence property values.

Professor Robert Inman (1978) was able to combine these findings into a simulation model that predicts the outcomes of a variety of reform proposals. Inman evaluated these outcomes according to three social welfare functions and then ranked the policies under each set of social values.

Two areas of investigation should be given high priority in future economic research on school finance: First, we must try to resolve the differences among the various estimates of the tax price elasticity of expenditures per pupil. Second, we must know how sensitive results such as Inman's are to the assumptions about behavioral responses and social values.

APPENDIXES

The process of designing a new school finance system involves a large number of technical issues in addition to the broad analytical and ethical issues discussed above. Alternative aid formulas, some of them quite complex, must be fed into a computer before the "best" formula can be identified. The school districts in any state are so diverse in their social and economic characteristics that it may be impossible to devise a simple system that sends just the right amount of financial aid to each locality.

Economists have played an important role in devising ways to deal with these complexities of school finance, and any accounting of the uses of economics in school finance analysis would be incomplete without some mention of the work on technical issues. Two major technical issues that have arisen in discussions of school finance reform have been subjected to extensive economic analysis: differences in the price of educational inputs among school districts and the special fiscal problems of central city school districts.

Appendix A discusses the first of these issues, differences in the price of educational inputs. Appendix B focuses on the set of problems usually referred to as municipal overburden. Appendix C treats the measurement of inequality. Because expenditure equalization is one (but *only* one) of the objectives of school finance reform, some measure or measures of inequality is an important tool in the evaluation of school finance systems.

157

Appendix A
COST-OF-EDUCATION INDEXES

THE CENTRAL PROBLEM: DIFFERENCES IN
SUPPLY CONDITIONS

Our objective in instituting a school finance reform is to alter the allocation of educational resources—teachers, classrooms, materials, and so on—among children. The only politically feasible way to do this while still maintaining the structure of decentralized management of education is to distribute state or federal aid dollars to school districts. So far in our discussions we have assumed that an allocation of dollars translates directly into an allocation of resources. We now relax this assumption and recognize that because the prices of educational resources vary among school districts, the same number of dollars may purchase different quantities of resources in different places.

The most obvious example of such price differences is land, and the differences are relatively easy to overcome. Central city land is much more expensive than suburban land which, in turn, is more valuable than rural land. It therefore will cost a central city school district more than a suburban or rural district to construct a school building of some given size and quality. If the state sent the same number of capital outlay dollars to all types of school districts with the intention of providing equal quality school buildings, that intention would be thwarted by differences in land prices. The problem of differential land prices can be remedied relatively easily in the design of school aid formulas. Differences in land prices and other construction costs are easy to find out, and districts may be reimbursed for allowable construction costs accordingly.

The subtler, and probably more troublesome, problem of differences in the price of teacher services is less easily remedied. A casual inspection of staff salaries in various school districts shows that apparently identical teachers are paid different amounts in different districts.

Why Teachers' Salaries Differ

One explanation for teacher salary differentials draws an analogy between the price of certain kinds of labor and the price of land. The reason for the high price of urban land is the fact that such land has many alternative uses, all of which generate high land rents. In some labor markets, college-educated workers have a large number of alternative occupations, each of which pays relatively high wages. In other labor markets, the public schools may be the only consumers of college-educated labor. Districts in the denser labor markets therefore might be forced to pay higher wages to compete successfully with other employers. Again, the same number of dollars sent to different districts would buy different quantities or qualities of teacher services, depending on conditions in the labor market in which the district happened to be located.

A second possible explanation for teacher salary differentials concerns the characteristics of jobs in different districts. Teaching in central city schools may simply be a more difficult job than teaching in suburban schools; if so, teachers with alternative job opportunities might insist on higher salaries before they would be willing to take central city teaching jobs. Central city districts then would be forced either to pay higher salaries to teachers of similar quality or to accept a lower quality work force at the same salaries paid by suburban districts.

If these explanations are sound and if the resulting differences in the prices of educational inputs are substantial, then some corrections should be made in aid formulas. Unfortunately, however, the design of such corrections has proved to be highly problematic. Some of the problems involved in the construction of cost-of-education indexes can be illustrated with a series of supply and demand diagrams.

To take the simplest problem first. Suppose that all teachers are of equal quality. Suppose further that the number of individuals willing to accept jobs as teachers in some school district increases as salaries increase, while the number of teachers the district wishes to hire decreases with the salary. Under these assumptions the local market for teachers can be illustrated as a supply and demand graph, as shown in Figure A–1.

Within the context of Figure A–1, different districts may pay different salaries to identical teachers because either the supply conditions or the demand conditions may vary. Consider two districts: *U*, an urban district, and *R*, a district in a suburban ring. Teaching in *U* is a harder job than teaching in *R*, and, to make matters worse, there are more high-paying alternative jobs for college graduates in *U* than in *R*. This means that at any given salary, fewer people will be willing to work as teachers in *U* than in *R*. Assume, finally, that the demand for teachers is identical in the two districts, as shown in Figure A–2. We can see from the diagram that under these circumstances district *U* will hire fewer teachers at a higher salary than district *R*.

Figure A–1. Supply and demand for teachers in a single school district

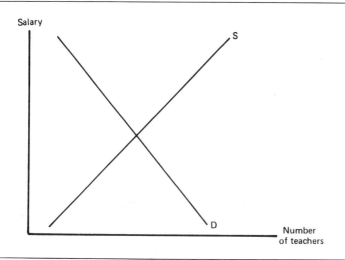

Figure A–2.   Identical demand and two supply curves

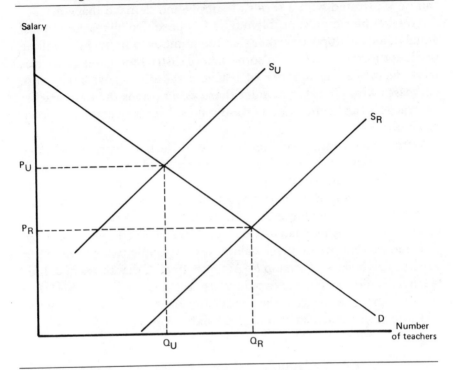

Now consider the case where demands differ among communities, but the supply conditions in each district are identical. Assume that for some reason—higher median income, lower tax price, or stronger preference for education—District A will demand more teachers at any given salary level than District B. These conditions are illustrated in Figure A–3. District A will hire more teachers at a higher salary than District B.

Note, however, that such a situation is not sustainable as an equilibrium if the two districts are in the same labor market. Since, by assumption, all teachers are identical, teachers in District B will not be satisfied with their lower salaries and will want to get jobs in District A. The supply of teachers to A will shift to the right and that to B will shift to the left. Salaries will adjust until all identical teachers receive the same salary, P*, the only sustainable equilibrium, as illustrated in Figure A–3. If the districts are in different labor market areas, the salary differential might be sustained.

Figure A–3. Identical supply, two demand curves, and supply curves shifting in response

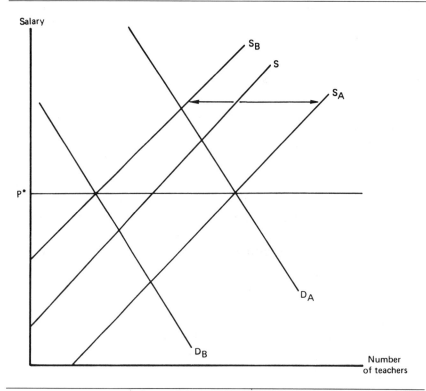

Differences in teachers' salaries, therefore, may reflect either or both of two sets of circumstances, one related to determinants of supply, the other to determinants of demand. The problem described in this appendix refers only to differences in supply conditions. Why should only supply-side factors constitute a problem? Suppose that we simply send more aid money to school districts where teacher salaries are higher. If we did so, we would be compensating places like District U, which are faced with unfavorable supply conditions, but we would also be sending more money to high-demand districts, like A, which are already relatively advantaged.

We want some way to isolate the supply-driven salary differences from demand-driven differences. This requirement defines the empirical task facing anyone who wishes to construct what analysts call a cost-of-education index. Several economists have undertaken this task and have proposed a number of analytical methodologies and results that lead to indexes. However, the process is conceptually complex, and the results are not yet widely accepted.

Teachers' Unions

A basic conceptual quandary must be resolved before we can justify the use of cost-of-education indexes and go on to describe the state of the art of cost-of-education-index construction. It may be that many parts of the country have substantial numbers of unemployed teachers. That is, a number of individuals may be qualified to teach and would take jobs in the public schools at current salary levels, but because of an insufficient demand for teacher services are either unemployed or have taken other jobs.

In the standard competitive model of labor markets, the one we have used to analyze the cost-of-education problem, such a situation could not arise. The presence of an unemployed work force would depress salary levels to the point where everyone willing to take a teaching job at the equilibrium wage rate would be so employed. However, the actual market for teachers may not work in this way.

In most states, public school teachers are permitted to form unions and to bargain collectively with local school authorities for contracts setting wages and working conditions. Organized teachers may be able to thwart the tendency of wages to drop in markets where unemployment is high. If this is the case, then we must look elsewhere than to differences in supply or demand conditions for our explanation of why the salaries of apparently identical teachers vary among school districts.

Within the context of a noncompetitive model, salaries are higher in districts where the current work force of teachers is better organized or more militant or where union officials are better negotiators than local school managers. Such circumstances would remove much of the justification for the inclusion of a cost-of-education index in the school aid formula. Compensating districts where teachers' salaries are high would remove the incentive for district managers to bargain as hard as they might to keep salaries down.

Although a state legislature might favor higher salaries for teachers across the board as a mechanism for attracting more able people to this profession over the long run, this issue differs from that of trying to insure that state aid formulas distribute educational resource purchasing power instead of raw dollars.

To what extent teacher markets are competitive or noncompetitive is a matter of judgment. If they are competitive and if supply conditions vary among school districts, then an attempt to design cost-of-education indexes is worthwhile. If these markets are predominantly noncompetitive, then cost differentials are probably a less important issue than they seem.

THE EMPIRICAL PROBLEM

We now return to the assumption that teacher markets are sufficiently competitive. Our task is to identify the portion of salary differentials among school districts that is atttributable to differences in the supply of teaching services. In other words, we want to weed out of the observed interdistrict variation in salaries all of the nonsupply-side effects.

Teachers' salaries vary with three broad categories of factors: the personal characteristics that determine the quality of teaching services that the individual teacher provides, the aggregate supply curve of teachers to the district in which he or she works, and the aggregate demand for teachers by the district. To isolate the supply-side effects on salaries, we must build a model that includes all of these classes of effects.

The first step in devising a cost-of-education index (more properly, an index of prices of teaching services) is to account for the fact that not all teachers are of identical quality. In our simple analysis of the cost differential problem, we assumed that teachers were identical and therefore were able to draw a single supply curve for each district. This assumption is unrealistic because each teacher is unique. The personnel office of a school district actually faces a large number of potential teachers, each with personal and professional characteristics and each willing to work in the district for any salary above some level. Although a model of teacher behavior that accounted for a wide variety of individual differences would be too complex to analyze, the assumption that all teachers are the same is too simple. Still, to compare prices among districts we must compare similar teachers.

Most researchers confronted with this problem use "hedonic regression techniques." This methodology assumes that the quality of a teacher can be represented by some linear combination of observable personal characteristics. Among the characteristics that might contribute or detract from quality are age (X_1), years of experience (X_2), years of postgraduate education (X_3), verbal ability (X_4), and so on. How much each of these characteristics contributes or detracts from teacher quality is determined by how much districts, on the average, are willing to pay for one more "unit" of each characteristic. If supply and demand characteristics for all types of teachers were the same in all school districts, we could obtain estimates of the perceived value of each of those characteristics by running a regression of the following form:

$$\text{Salary} = \beta_0 + \beta_1 X_1 + \beta_2 X_2 + \beta_3 X_3 + \beta_4 X_4 + \ldots \quad (A-1)$$

where our observations would be individual teachers, their characteristics, and their salaries, and where β could represent, say, the degree to which each characteristic contributed to teacher quality. Alternatively, we might estimate a similar equation using average values of salaries and characteristics for a sample of school districts. Of course, the entire discussion in Appendix A is posited on the supposition that supply and demand conditions vary among districts; therefore, equation $(A-1)$ could not be estimated on its own. Equation $(A-1)$ is actually part of a larger model of salary determination, the part that accounts for variation by quality of teaching services.

The next step is to model the determinants of a district's demand for teacher services. We have already noted some of the factors that might shift a district's demand curve for teachers. In general, districts that are able and willing to provide a relatively high level of educational services will demand relatively large numbers of teachers. Districts with high median incomes and low tax prices tend to provide the highest level of educational services. We can, therefore, expect that increases in median income (Y) and decreases in tax prices (t) will shift a district's demand for teachers to the right.

On the supply side, we have argued that high alternative wages for college graduates and more difficult working conditions tend to reduce the supply of teachers to a district. These two factors may be measured by variables representing average wages for college graduates other than teachers in the labor market in which the district is located, w; the mean socioeconomic status of the student population, *ses*; the degree of violence in the schools, *v*; and other indicators of working conditions, *c*.

Our supposition is that teacher characteristics, demand conditions, and supply conditions act simultaneously and independently to determine teacher salaries. This assumption can be expressed in a regression equation.

$$\text{Mean Salary} = \beta_0 + \beta_1 X_1 + \beta_2 X_2 + \beta_3 X_3 + \beta_4 X_4 + \beta_5 Y$$
$$+ \beta_6 t + \beta_7 w + \beta_8 ses + \beta_9 v + \beta_{10} c \qquad \text{(A-2)}$$

Estimates of equations such as (A–2) might enable us to isolate the supply-side effects and therefore to compute a cost-of-education index. The computation would proceed as follows. We want to compare supply conditions in any given district with those of the average district in the state. To do so, we construct the following ratio:

$$I_j = \frac{\beta_7 w + \beta_8 ses + \beta_9 v + \beta_{10} c}{\beta_7 W + \beta_8 SES + \beta_9 V + \beta_{10} C}$$

where the variables in the numerator (*w, v, ses,* and so on) are for a specific district, those in the denominator (*W, V, SES,* and so on) are the averages for those variables for all of the districts in the state, and I_j is the cost-of-education index for district *j*. $I_j = 1.10$ would mean that because of adverse supply conditions, district *j* was forced to pay 10 percent more than the average district to attract teachers of average quality. The observed salary differential between district *j* and the state average might be, say, 20 percent, but these hypothetical estimates would indicate that only about half of the gross difference, 10 percent, was attributable to adverse supply conditions.

The index I_j could be used quite simply to adjust a basic school finance formula for interdistrict cost-of-education differentials. The state would simply send district *j* 10 percent more than what it was entitled to under the basic formula. Since the average district would have an index of 1.00, about half the districts would have indexes of less than 1.00 and about half would have indexes of more than 1.00. The total amount of money the state distributed through the school aid formula therefore would be the same, whether or not a cost adjustment index was used. The effect would be a distribution of purchasing power instead of raw dollars.

THE VALIDITY OF A COST-OF-EDUCATION INDEX

The reader should be sufficiently familiar by now with the potential unreliability of even the most sophisticated economic analysis to suspect that this optimistic assessment of the usefulness of existing cost-of-education indexes is overdrawn. Indeed it is. We already have mentioned one fundamental, unresolved problem: Teacher markets may not be competitive, and therefore much of the justification for the use of these indexes may be unfounded. Two further difficulties undermine the validity of existing indexes, even if the justification for their use is accepted.

First, no empirical study will be able to identify all of the differences in the quality of teachers among school districts. The measurable attributes of teachers—age, experience, level of education, and verbal skills—do not capture many of the most important elements of good teaching. To see why this should create a problem with respect to index creation, consider two districts with identical salary schedules. Both districts pay apparently identical teachers the same salaries. Suppose further that teaching is an easier or more rewarding job in one district than in another. Assume, finally, that some characteristics associated with teacher quality are neither accounted for in the salary schedule nor observable in the statistical sense, but are known to the two districts' personnel offices. Under these circumstances the personnel officers will offer jobs to the best teachers first. These best teachers will take jobs in the better district and the other district will have to hire the worst teachers.

It would, in fact, cost more for the less favored district to attract teachers of any given quality, but this difference will not be detected by the methodology described above.

Second, up to this point we have assumed that there is some obvious distinction between variables that influence the demand for and those that determine the supply of teacher services. In fact, no such clear demarcation is possible. Consider the case of the median income of school district residents, which we identified in equation (A–2) as influencing the demand for teachers. However, we know that all workers (teachers and others) tend to receive higher pay for similar work in areas where median income is higher. It is difficult, therefore, to separate the effects of median income and alternative wages on teacher salaries, and it is uncertain whether the coefficient on the income term (β_5) is measuring a supply-side effect or a demand-side effect. The effects of mean pupil *SES* may be similar. The parents of hard-to-educate children might demand more teaching services than the parents of higher *SES* children. This parental demand might be reflected in district demand, especially since low-*SES* children draw federal compensatory education revenues into the district. Does low *SES* increase demand and therefore raise salaries, or does it decrease supply and hence raise salaries? We cannot say for sure.

The lack of a clear distinction between supply and demand effects renders our index values uncertain. If we judge that *SES* and income influence supply but not demand, our index would be

$$I_j = \frac{\beta_7 w + \beta_8 ses + \beta_9 v + \beta_{10} c}{\beta_7 W + \beta_8 SES + \beta_9 V + \beta_{10} C}$$

If, however, we made the opposite judgment—that income and *SES* influence only demand, and not supply—the alternative index would be

$$I'_j = \frac{\beta_7 w + \beta_{10} c}{\beta_7 W + \beta_{10} C}$$

If experiments like this were undertaken using actual regression results from equations such as (A−2), we would expect to find that I_j and I'_j tend to differ for some districts. The basic trends in values for I, with the central city having the highest indexes and rural districts the lowest, are expected regardless of the demarcation of supply and demand factors. However, the actual allocation of school aid dollars among districts might differ, depending on which specification was adopted. Since the distinction has a shaky analytical basis, so do the indexes derived from that demarcation.

One final caveat is that the use of cost-of-education indexes might create adverse incentives for school districts. Suppose we found that a high level of violence in schools reduces the supply of teachers to a district and therefore raises the price. The districts with a high incidence of school violence would receive relatively more state aid. This might reduce the incentive for districts to adopt costly programs to reduce violence in the schools.

SUMMARY

The prices of educational inputs may vary among school districts. If they do, then states wanting to redistribute educational services and not just raw dollars among school districts will have to adjust their aid formulas to reflect the price differentials. Both supply and demand factors influence the prices of educational inputs, but the argument for adjusting aid formulas really applies only to differences in prices attributable to supply-side effects.

The empirical problem involved in devising a cost-of-education index (or an index of prices of educational inputs) is to identify the influence of supply-side factors on the prices faced by school district managers. The difficulty of this empirical undertaking stems, first, from the difficulty of distinguishing factors affecting supply from those influencing demand. Arbitrary distinctions between these two classes of factors have led to essentially arbitrary indexes. Second, it is difficult to measure the quality of teachers. It is important to do so, however, because we want to compare the prices of essentially identical inputs. However, the qualities that make a good teacher are imperfectly related to the observable characteristics of teachers. For these reasons, no completely satisfactory methodology for computing cost-of-education indexes has yet been devised.

All of this is not to say that cost-of-education indexes ought not to be adopted as aid formula elements. The judgment that the problems discussed at the beginning of Appendix A are real and important could certainly be legitimate. This caveat tells us only that the state of the cost-index art has not reached the point where a simple, definitive methodology can be blindly adopted by all policymakers.

Appendix B
THE SPECIAL PROBLEM
OF CITIES:
MUNICIPAL OVERBURDEN

Large city[1] school districts command more than their proportionate share of the attention of school finance activists and policymakers for several reasons. First, large urban districts serve large proportions of children who are of special social welfare concern: the poor, the handicapped, non-English speakers, and low achievers. Second, all studies of differences in the price of educational inputs among school districts conclude that big city districts pay more than others for identical educational resources.

Third, most large cities do not fit well into the traditional formulation of the general school finance problem. The summary statistics, which characterize the relative financial conditions of suburban or rural school districts quite well, do not account adequately for big city school district fiscal circumstances. In most states, large cities enjoy relatively large property tax bases per pupil and set relatively low tax rates for educational purposes. Central cities sometimes spend considerably more per pupil than the average district, because of the higher level of state and federal categorical aid they receive. If these summary statistics are all that enter any new school aid formula, then cities will receive proportionately less new aid than other types of districts.

1. Throughout this appendix, large city school districts will be referred to as central city, large city, or urban districts. These terms may be taken to refer to the central cities of most standard metropolitan statistical areas.

171

Finally, big city governments generally spend more per capita on nonschool public services and tax at higher rates for general local government services than other jurisdictions. This observation has led some analysts to hypothesize that noneducational demands on urban tax bases may limit the resources available for educational services, a condition that they call "municipal overburden." According to the hypothesis, the higher the nonschool local tax rate, the lower the local revenues available for education.

The general framework for economic analysis of school finance issues developed up to this point seems adequate for dealing with three of the four special urban problems listed above. Social welfare concern for disadvantaged groups necessarily will send more money to urban districts. State-of-the-art cost indexes will have the same effect. If our approach to school finance reform is modified with these factors in mind, then we need not worry about the tendency of equalization mechanisms to direct aid away from needy urban districts.

The fourth potential problem—municipal overburden—remains. If cities are overburdened, but this condition is not accounted for in our aid formula, then central city school districts will receive suboptimal payments. In other words, corrections for the kinds of students served by these districts and for adverse supply conditions may not account for the total severity of the problems facing these districts.

To correct for the potential problem of municipal overburden, state school aid formulas ought to incorporate an overburden factor that would send relatively more aid to districts where nonschool local taxes are high. Michigan already includes a specific municipal overburden factor in its school finance formula, and the New York Supreme Court has ruled that state's school finance system unconstitutional, partly because it fails to account for municipal overburden. At the same time, several very large cities are experiencing severe fiscal stress.

Despite the seeming simplicity of the analytic argument behind the municipal overburden hypothesis as it is usually stated, the hypothesis has never been systematically confirmed. If the hypothesis is not valid, inclusion of an overburden factor in an aid formula could lead to a misallocation of funds. We want to know, then, whether the hypothesis is true and, if so, whether it precisely identifies the fiscal problems of large urban school districts.

THE VALIDITY OF THE
OVERBURDEN HYPOTHESIS

The overburden hypothesis has not been confirmed, because the evidence presented to support it is open to other, sometimes contradictory, interpretations. An examination of some alternative explanations for relative values of central city fiscal variables indicates why the hypothesis has not been sustained.

Consider first the possibility that high levels of public expenditures are simply one of the costs associated with city life. Dense populations increase the incidence of fires and crimes; public health and sanitation require more care; heavy traffic increases the cost of maintaining a road network. At the same time, there are substantial benefits to living in cities. Central city residents commute shorter distances to work and to shop, and city life offers cultural opportunities that are less accessible to residents of suburbs or rural areas. If the benefits of city living justify the costs, then it seems unreasonable to take high nonschool expenditures and taxes as evidence that central city residents are overburdened.

The costs and benefits of city life may not, however, be in balance. If low-income people or minorities are confined to central cities by suburban zoning regulations and racial discrimination, the costs that these groups bear may outweigh the benefits. However, to show that central city residents bear an unfair burden of local public expenditure, one first must demonstrate that they would not live in the city except for artificial constraints. In some metropolitan areas poor people have housing options in the suburbs; in others, they do not. Establishing the presence of some net overburden, then, is more complicated in analytical undertaking than the simple hypothesis would suggest.

Pursuing a different line of reasoning, one can show that the relative values of central city fiscal indicators easily could mean exactly the opposite of what proponents of the municipal overburden hypothesis contend. Central city tax bases include a much higher proportion of nonresidential property than those of suburban jurisdictions. The burden of taxes on commercial and industrial property is either passed forward to consumers of these firms' output or backward to the owners of the firms themselves. In either case, a substantial proportion of the burden of central city taxes is borne by nonresidents.

Furthermore, much of the housing in central cities is renter-occupied, and at least a portion of the tax on such property is borne by absentee landlords. Again, part of the burden of central city taxation may be passed on to nonresidents. In other words, central city voters are faced with a much lower tax price than suburban or rural voters. In response, central city residents may be expected to support higher levels of spending. The higher expenditures observed in central cities, therefore, may reflect not a relative overburden but the relative fiscal advantages of central cities.

The final problem with the municipal overburden hypothesis as it usually has been stated is that its proponents have not been clear about the institutional interaction between school spending and general municipal spending. What public choice mechanism would dictate that high nonschool spending left less to be spent by schools? We could not draw such a conclusion within the context of the median voter model. The median voter would choose a level of spending for general government and for schools independently, and these would be no more closely related than any other two categories of consumption.

Models could, of course, be devised to predict inverse relationship between school and nonschool spending, but most such models have tended to be ad hoc and unrelated to any more general theory of local public choice. Furthermore, the empirical hypothesis of an inverse relationship between nonschool and school spending has never received more than very weak statistical confirmation (Brazer 1974). If the municipal overburden hypothesis were true, then we would expect to find nonschool spending associated with a significant negative coefficient in a regression equation predicting expenditures per pupil. When analysts have estimated such equations, the nonschool expenditure term has never been associated with a strongly negative coefficient.

The traditional municipal overburden hypothesis, then, does not give the impression of having much a priori or empirical validity. Still, we observe that some cities are in severe fiscal straits and that few other types of jurisdictions are in as bad shape. Certainly, the schools in fiscally stressed cities appear to be suffering along with the rest of the public sector. Any state school finance plan that assumed that these cities were capable of raising more local revenues or even of maintaining their current levies would certainly be suspect. We are left, therefore, with the problem of identifying cities that are experiencing stress. Higher-than-average expenditures or taxes are not the distinguishing characteristic, since these indicators may signify too many different underlying conditions. What characteristics, then, distinguish cities in fiscal stress?

THE FISCAL STRESS CRITERION

At least one set of circumstances would render the municipal overburden argument valid. If a governmental jurisdiction had fixed revenues to allocate to all public services, then any money spent on noneducational activities would leave that much less available for schools. If the educational services provided by that jurisdiction were inadequate by the state's social welfare standard, then the state would have to induce the locality to reduce its spending on other public services, or it would have to send more state aid to the local school district. In any case, it would be unreasonable to expect the locality to devote more local resources to education without some reduction in other public expenditure categories.

When might a jurisdiction be faced with fixed local revenues? Certainly in the short run, the amount of revenue could not be fixed. The total resources theoretically available to a local government in any given year are equal to all personal income of residents (above some subsistence level), all of the profits of local firms, and all rents paid to local property owners. Since no jurisdiction is currently drawing this much revenue from local taxpayers, any locality could increase total local revenues in any given year.

In the long run, however, households and firms could respond to high taxes in a locality by moving elsewhere. Indeed, if any jurisdiction attempted to tax away all local income, profits, and rent, we would expect no one to remain there after a few years. Of course, the jurisdiction would use its tax revenues to provide public services, which would be expected to make the community a better place to locate. However, a local government can tax itself at too high a rate, provide too high a level of public services, and thereby induce resident firms and households to leave.

In the final analysis, therefore, the level of revenues that a jurisdiction can raise may be fixed. Revenues could be increased at any time by raising tax rates, but this tax increase would drive out enough potential taxpayers that future revenue-raising capacity would be diminished. In a sense, a community that taxed at this rate would be borrowing from future revenues to finance current services. Further tax increases would decrease long-run revenues, so that future expenditures would have to decrease, unless some higher level of government came to the rescue.

This condition, called "fiscal stress," may validate the municipal overburden argument.

Consider two communities, A and B. Jurisdiction A is experiencing fiscal stress; community B is not. B could raise tax rates now with no appreciable effect on future revenues and therefore could be expected to maintain a higher level of expenditures on schools and other services indefinitely. Community A could not. A state government could reasonably expect community B to raise additional local revenues for schools in response to an inducement, such as a matching grant, without decreasing nonschool expenditures. It could not reasonably expect the same of community A. School finance conditions in the two communities are therefore different in ways that may not be adequately reflected in such statistics as assessed value per pupil or local tax rates.

Fiscally stressed communities are not readily identifiable until some financial crisis draws our attention. High taxes and high expenditures alone do not tell the whole story, because what we want is an assessment of the current rate of taxation relative to the maximum level the jurisdiction can tax itself without ultimately diminishing revenues. Identifying the ideal measure of fiscal stress therefore involves estimating the long-term revenue-maximizing tax rate and level of public expenditures. So far this task has exceeded our ability.

We can nevertheless identify the characteristics of communities likely to experience fiscal stress. Specifically, jurisdictions characterized by low general economic growth rates and relatively high tax rates are more likely than other types of communities to suffer stress. An analogy between political jurisdictions and households should indicate why this is so.

A jurisdiction that issues no bonds but taxes itself above its revenue-maximizing tax rate is borrowing against its own future revenues; that is, it is spending revenues now at the expense of future spending. This is the essence of borrowing. Under certain circumstances, borrowing against future income is a reasonable economic choice.

A household that expects its income to rise may choose, by borrowing, to enjoy some of the benefits of that future income before it is actually received. If income is growing rapidly, the household need not be especially concerned if, in any given year, expenditures exceed income. Annual spending may continue to increase even after the household begins to repay its debts.

On the other hand, a household with constant or declining income would not have the same opportunity to borrow. With constant income, any increase in spending over income must be matched by a decrease in spending below current income in the future. If a household with decreasing income borrows, future spending must decrease faster than income to repay the debt. Although the analogy between a household and a city is far from exact, the same basic logic applies to both.

The equivalent of annual income for a city is its tax base. If the tax base is growing at a rapid rate, the city can levy high taxes at any time, forgoing some small portion of its potential tax-base growth, and still expect annual spending to increase, or at least to remain constant. With a stable or declining tax base, however, high spending is more likely to require a decrease in future spending.

The tax base, in turn, reflects the level of economic activity within the jurisdiction. A low or negative economic growth rate coupled with a high tax rate characterizes fiscally stressed communities.

The municipal overburden argument has come full circle. Cities in the northeast and northcentral regions of the United States appear to suffer the lowest economic growth rate. Conditions in these cities raised the concern that originally led to the municipal overburden hypothesis. This hypothesis was seen to be less than convincing on conceptual and theoretical grounds. Nevertheless, a circuitous route from that hypothesis has led us back to the conclusion that some cities—specifically, those suffering fiscal stress—may deserve more state school aid than they apparently would receive purely on the grounds of equalization.

Having made the fiscal stress argument, we know three things about urban school finance that we did not know before. First, we have identified the conditions under which the fiscal condition of urban school districts presents a special problem. High taxes and expenditures alone do not necessarily signal overburden. Instead, we must focus on observed tax rates relative to the maximum level of revenues the jurisdiction could sustain. Second, we have observed the difficulty of determining with certainty whether a city is likely to experience fiscal stress. Finally, we have shown that the cities most likely to experience stress are those with low economic growth rates.

We do not yet know, however, the quantitative characteristics of fiscal stress—how low the growth rate and how high the tax rate must be before a fiscal crisis becomes inevitable. We do know that progress in research on urban fiscal conditions will require an empirical estimate of the maximum rate at which a city could tax, given the growth rate of its local economy, and not expect to become bankrupt.

SUMMARY

Many of the problems discussed elsewhere in this study are more severe in central city than in other types of school districts. Large cities may, however, have an additional problem, diagnosed as municipal overburden. According to the municipal overburden hypothesis, because they generally spend more per capita and tax themselves at higher rates to support nonschool public services than do other jurisdictions, large cities have less to spend on education. Because cities may be more severely constrained in their ability to raise school revenues, the argument continues, special consideration of urban districts ought to be built into any state's school aid formula.

This argument has been examined and found wanting, because the observed data—higher than average spending per capita and nonschool tax rates—are open to other, sometimes contradictory, interpretations. The conclusion that high nonschool spending limits school spending is only one of many that may be drawn from the data.

An alternative way of looking at the urban school finance problem is to focus on fiscal stress and fiscal crises. If a city that has been spending more than it can maintain over a long period faces a crisis and is forced to reduce total spending, the city's schools will suffer along with other local public services. Although it is difficult to predict which cities are likely to experience crisis, we know that a slow tax-base growth rate and a high tax rate characterize cities with a high crisis potential.

Appendix C
THE MEASUREMENT
OF EQUALITY

This study has made much of the multiplicity of objectives toward which school finance reform might lead. In Chapter 7, these goals were subsumed under three categories: aggregate, subjective household well-being and its distribution, resource equality among students, and school district institutional integrity.

With regard to the objective of resource equality, we argued that the rights protected under the Fourteenth Amendment and similar provisions in state constitutions could be interpreted as requiring that any deviation from strict resource equality be justifiable. In other words, expenditure inequality must be considered costly in terms of social welfare, and this cost must be matched by some social benefit.

EXPENDITURE EQUALITY AS A GOAL
OF REFORM

In evaluating any change in school finance systems, therefore, one factor that must be taken into account is the effect of the reform on the degree of expenditure inequality. To determine whether expenditures have or will become more equal and by how much, we need measures of inequality.

179

Before discussing several alternative measures of inequality, it is important to point out the danger involved in the measurement of this particular characteristic of school finance systems. Resource equalization is only one goal of reform. This particular objective may be viewed as relatively important or unimportant, depending on one's subjective values. Those who place high subjective value on household well-being or school district institutional integrity may assign little relative importance to expenditure equality.

This multiplicity of value orientations would not present a problem except that expenditure inequality is much easier to measure than any of the other reasonable goals of school finance reform. Data on expenditures are readily available in most states, and the conceptual basis for the measurement of inequality are well developed. The same cannot be said for the goals of household well-being or school district integrity.

The danger is that it is easy to focus our attention on the single objective for which measures are available at the expense of less readily quantifiable goals. Too narrow a focus in policy design and evaluation can lead to poor policymaking.

The following discussion, therefore, is presented with the caveat that expenditure equalization is only one objective of school finance reform and quite legitimately may be assigned very little importance.

Equality—or inequality—may be measured in several different ways, but the basic idea behind each of them is to enable us to compare distributions (of income, expenditures per pupil, educational resources, tax-burdens, etc.) among economic units (states, school districts, schools, households, pupils, etc.).

To give concreteness to our discussion, we will consider the distribution of expenditures per pupil among the school districts in a hypothetical state, using the data presented in Table C–1.

We want to answer the following questions: Did the equality of expenditure distribution increase between 1970 and 1980? Did equality increase more between 1975 and 1980 than between 1970 and 1975? The oversimplified answer to both questions, of course, is that expenditures remained unequal throughout the period, because equality is an absolute relationship. School reform, however, does not strive for perfect expenditure equality, which may not be obtainable or even desirable. Reform aims, rather, at movements in the direction of equality. It is useful, therefore, to have measures that indicate the

Table C–1. Hypothetical school district expenditure data

District	Expenditures per Pupil		
	1970	1975	1980
A	800	1000	1200
B	500	1000	1300
C	700	1500	2000
D	1000	1800	2100
E	500	900	1000

direction and magnitude of movements toward or away from perfect equality.

Several measures of equality are commonly used, because each measures a different aspect of the distribution. Equality measures (or indexes of equality) differ in several respects. Some report a decrease in inequality whenever expenditures in a high-spending district decrease or expenditures in a low-spending district increase. Other indexes register no change in inequality when some such changes in the distribution take place. Some indexes value equally all increases in expenditure by districts below the mean and all decreases by districts above the mean. Others show larger decreases in inequality when very low-spending districts increase their expenditures than when districts below but close to the mean increase theirs by a like amount. Still other indexes may treat changes in different parts of the distribution differently, depending on how the index is calculated.

If all districts changed their expenditures by a constant proportion (say, 10 percent) or by a fixed amount (say, $200 per pupil) some indexes would register an increase in equality, some a decrease, and some no change at all.

Some measures are complete; others are not. That is, given any two distributions, some measures indicate whether the two distributions differ in the degree of inequality and, if so, which is the more equal distribution. Such measures of equality are said to be complete. Incomplete measures cannot be used to gauge the relative inequality of some pairs of distributions.

These distinctions are more than conceptual curiosities. Each index measures different aspects of equality. Just which aspect of equality is important is a matter of personal judgment. Who is to say whether equality rises or falls when all districts increase their spending per pupil by a constant proportional amount or by a uniform amount? Does an increase in spending by the lowest-spending district reduce inequality more than would a similar increase by a district just below the mean? Some would say yes and others would say no. Those who hold different positions on these questions would evaluate the difference in inequality between two distributions differently.

The different measures, each reflecting different judgments as to the importance of various aspects of equality, evaluate any given change in a distribution differently (as the sample computations in Table C–2 indicate). For this reason, analysts can do no more than to compute several equality measures, report the findings, and allow the consumer to focus on the index that most closely conforms to his own judgments about what constitutes equality.

SOME EQUALITY INDEXES

We discuss below only a few of the inequality indexes that have appeared in the extensive literature on this topic. Our criteria for selecting measures for this presentation were ease of conceptual comprehensibility and frequency of use in school finance literature (Berne and Stiefel 1979; Inman 1978).

Range and Restricted Range

The range is simply the difference between the highest and lowest observation. The restricted range excludes outliers, comparing, say, the district spending more than 75 percent of all other districts with the district spending less than 75 percent of all other districts. For our hypothetical data, the range is $500 in 1970, $900 in 1975, and $1,100 in 1980. According to this measure, expenditure inequality rose over the decade. If we use the range as our index, only changes in spending by the lowest-spending or the highest-spending districts will register as changes in inequality. Constant proportional increases in all districts' spending will increase inequality; uniform dollar changes in all districts will not affect the index. The range is a complete measure in that the equality of any two distributions can be compared.

Variance and Related Measures

Variance, a familiar statistical concept, measures the average squared differences between each observation and the mean of the distribution. The formula for computing the variance is

$$V = \frac{1}{n} \sum_{i=1}^{n} (X_i - \overline{X})^2$$

The variance is a complete equality measure. Any increase in spending by a lower-than-average district or any decrease by a higher-than-average district registers a decrease in inequality. Changes in spending by districts at the extremes of the distribution affect this equality measure more than do changes close to the distribution mean. Proportionate increases in all district expenditures increase inequality as measured by the variance; uniform dollar increases have no effect on equality.

Three commonly used statistics relate closely to the variance. The standard deviation—that is, the square root of the variance—shares all of the properties of the variance itself as a measure of equality. The variance of the logarithms is computed by taking the natural logarithm of each observation and then calculating the variance using these transformed data. The properties of the variance of the logarithms are the same as those of the variance, except that increases in expenditures by the lowest-spending districts decrease inequality by much more than similar reductions in expenditures by high-spending districts. The variance of the logarithms also produces an equality measure that does not change value when expenditures in all districts increase by an equal proportion.

The coefficient of variation (CV) is simply the variance divided by the mean of the distribution. It shares all of the characteristics of the variance, except that the CV does not change when expenditures increase everywhere by an equal proportion.

The Lorenz Curve and Gini Coefficient

These two closely related measures are best explained by starting with the Lorenz curve. We draw two axes, one representing the percentage of total expenditures per pupil and the other the percentage of school districts. If all districts spent exactly the same amount per pupil, then 20 percent of the districts would account for 20 percent of total expenditures per pupil, 40 percent of the districts would account for 40 percent of the expenditures, and so on. The graph traced by a perfectly equal distribution would look like line *OD* in Figure C–1 and, in fact, is called the line of perfect equality.

To determine the existence of inequality among the school districts, we array them along the horizontal axis in ascending order of expenditures and plot the percentage of total expenditures per pupil. Taking the hypothetical 1970 data in Table C–1, consider, first, District *E*. It is one of five, or 20 percent of the total number of districts. Its expenditure of $500 per pupil, however, represents only 14 percent of the total expenditure per pupil of ($800 + $700 + $1000 + $500

Figure C–1. Line of perfect equality and Lorenz curve (based on data from Table C–1)

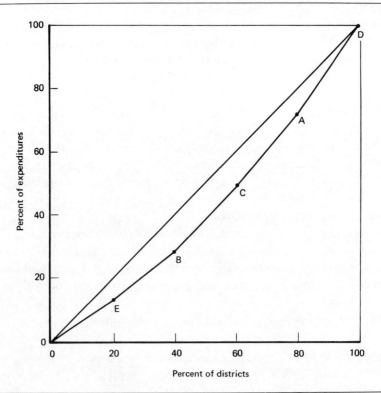

=) $3500. This combination of 20 percent of the districts and 14 percent of expenditures is represented by point E in Figure C–1. Districts E and B together, in turn, represent 40 percent of all districts and 28 percent of expenditures. This combination is represented by point B in Figure C–1. The process is repeated until all districts are accounted for. Inequality among districts would cause the curve traced by the distribution to bow out from the line of perfect equality, as does $OEBCAD$, the Lorenz curve for the hypothetical 1970 distribution, in Figure C–1. The further this curve bows out from the line of perfect equality, the more unequal the distribution.

Using similar graphs, we show why the Lorenz curve is an "incomplete" index of inequality. Suppose we want to compare the distributions A and B illustrated in Figure C–2. Because curve A lies entirely inside curve B, we conclude that distribution A is more equal than distribution B. If we want to compare distributions B and C, however, we can make no such definitive statement. Because the Lorenz curves cross, we cannot state which of the two distributions is more equal.

Figure C–2.   Illustration of incompleteness of Lorenz curve

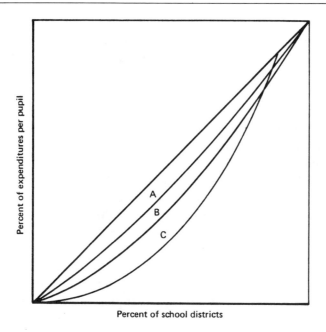

Percent of expenditures per pupil

A

B

C

Percent of school districts

Figure C–3.   Line of perfect equality, Lorenz curve, and Gini coefficient (ratio of area *A* to area *A* + *B*)

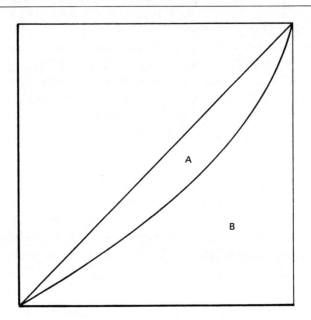

Any increase in spending by a district anywhere below the median and any decrease by a district anywhere above the median registers as a decrease in inequality by the Lorenz curve measure. Neither proportional nor uniform changes in expenditures in all districts has any effect on equality by this measure.

To obtain a more complete index, the analyst may use the Gini coefficient to examine the areas defined by these curves. This coefficient is the ratio of the area between the Lorenz curve and the line of perfect equality and the total area below the line of total equality. In Figure C–3, the Gini coefficient is the ratio of area *A* to area *A* + *B*. The coefficient ranges, therefore, between the value zero, representing perfect equality, and one, indicating perfect inequality.

The Gini coefficient shares all of the properties of the Lorenz curve, except that the Gini coefficient of two distributions may be compared even when the Lorenz curves associated with those coefficients cross. The Gini coefficient is, therefore, a complete measure of equality.

The Atkinson Index

As noted above, some equality indexes register the same drop in inequality whenever spending in a district below the mean increases by some given dollar amount. Other indexes show that the drop in inequality is larger when one of the lowest-spending districts increases its expenditures than when a district close to but still below the mean increases expenditures by a like amount. That is, some measures value increases in spending at the low end of the distribution relatively more than increases at the middle or at the high end.

The Atkinson (1970) index has the advantage of allowing the analyst to specify beforehand the degree to which the equality index exhibits this characteristic of favoritism toward the low end of the distribution. That the Atkinson index exhibits this characteristic is not immediately obvious when one inspects its formula.

$$ A = 1 - \left[\sum_{i=1}^{n} \left(\frac{X_i}{\overline{X}} \right)^{1-E} \right]^{\frac{1}{1-E}} $$

E represents the degree to which the index will favor districts lower down in the distribution. If $E = 0$, then all districts are equally favored, and increases in spending by any district, rich or poor, will be valued equally. As E increases, Atkinson's index places increasing emphasis on the expenditures in the lowest-spending districts. If E is set at a very high value, the Atkinson index will compare distributions solely on the basis of expenditures in the lowest-spending district.

The Atkinson index is complete, and its value does not change with proportional or uniform increases in spending among districts. This measure differs from all others in that increases in the Atkinson index indicate decreases in inequality, while increases in the others indicate increases in inequality. Typically, an equality assessment using the Atkinson index presents the results of several different computations, each with a specific value for E.

The evaluation of the changes in inequality differ markedly among indexes. Table C–2, based on the hypothetical school district expenditure data given in Table C–1 (p. 181), shows that between 1970 and 1975, depending on the measure used, inequality increased by 240 percent (the variance), decreased by 45 percent (the Atkinson index, $E = 10$), or something in between. This disparity means that one's personal feelings about what constitutes equality or inequality matter.

An analyst who believes that gross dollar differences in expenditure between all school districts constitute the most important kind of inequality would choose the variance to measure inequality. Given this set of values, inequality has increased markedly over the decade. The analyst who believes that the existence of very low-spending districts is the most troublesome aspect of inequality and that the expenditure patterns among other districts matter less would adopt the second of the two Atkinson indexes in Table C–2. According to this value orientation, inequality decreased over the decade, because spending in the poorest district increased steadily.

One message of this appendix is that values matter and that analysts setting out to measure inequality should compute and present several alternative measures and explain which aspects of inequality are reflected in each measure. The second message, stated as strongly as

Table C–2.   Equality indexes based on hypothetical data in Table C–1

	Value of Index			Percent Change[a]	
	1970	1975	1980	1970–75	1975–80
Range	500	900	1100	+80	+22
Restricted range (excludes highest and lowest)	200	500	800	+150	+60
Variance	36,000	122,400	197,600	+240	+61
Variance of logarithms	.073	.073	.085	0	+16
Coefficient of variation	51.43	98.71	130	+92	+32
Gini coefficient	.15	.15	.16	0	+7
Atkinson's index (E = .05)	.99	.99	.99	0	0
Atkinson's index (E = 10)	4.42	6.39	11.19	+45	+75

[a]Increases in Atkinson's index indicate decreases in measured inequality. Increases in all other indexes indicate increases in measured inequality.

possible at the beginning of Appendix C, is that expenditure equality is only one of several reasonable objectives of school finance reform. The relative ease with which this particular outcome is measured should not distract us from the pursuit of all other objectives.

SUMMARY

The inequality exhibited by a distribution, for example, of expenditures per pupil among school districts, has several aspects. Which aspect or aspects one considers most worthy of alleviation by public policy is a matter of personal value judgment. Measures are available for evaluating several aspects of equality, but no single measure includes all aspects. Depending on which measure one chooses, either of two distributions may be reported as the more equal. Therefore, in any analysis of equality, several measures should be computed and reported, along with explicit descriptions of which aspect of equality is more important.

The reduction of inequality is only one objective of reform and may be considered of minor importance to many reformers. No evaluation of alternative school finance systems should be confined to reporting measures of equality.

GLOSSARY

Ad valorem tax: A tax that is proportional to the market value of a good.

Benefit principle: The belief that households should pay taxes to support a government activity in proportion to the benefit they derive from that activity.

Capitalization of taxes: The effect of taxes on the market value of the taxed good, especially in reference to capital assets (land, buildings, bonds, stocks, etc.).

Categorical aid (categorical programs): Intergovernmental aid to school districts to finance specific educational programs, usually serving specific types of pupils.

Coefficient: A numerical measure of the effect of an independent variable on a dependent variable.

Colinearity: An econometric problem that arises when two variables are such that when one is above its average value the other is almost always above (or below) its average value by a like proportion.

Constrained maximization: A mathematical problem-solving technique whereby the user chooses the values for a set of control variables (or instruments) so as to attain certain prespecified objectives, subject to a set of constraints.

Consumer surplus: The difference between the actual price of a good and what the consumer would be willing to pay for that good; the total subjective well-being experienced by households as a result of the consumption of some good.

Control variable: A variable whose value is set by the government.

Cost-of-education index: A number representing the cost to a school district of purchasing some prespecified combination of educational inputs (teachers, equipment, buildings, etc.) relative to the average cost of purchasing those inputs in all school districts.

Dead-weight loss: See **Excess burden.**

Demand curve: A set of points, each representing the quantity of a good that would be purchased at a given price.

Dependent variable: A variable whose value is determined by the relationships accounted for in a model.

Differential property tax: The portion of the property tax, as administered in the United States, which differs from location to location.

Discount rate: An interest rate.

Disposable income: Total income minus tax payments.

Econometrics: The application of statistical theory and methodology to predictive economic theory to add quantitative (empirical) content to the qualitative predictions generated by theory.

Elasticity (inelasticity): The responsiveness of one variable to another. Demand is price-inelastic, for example, if the quantity purchased changes very little when the price changes by a great deal.

Empirical: Based on observation or experience.

Equalization aid: Intergovernmental aid to school districts to reduce interdistrict disparities in either spending per pupil or local school tax rates.

Excess burden: The difference between the value of the total well-being lost through taxation and the value of the tax revenues collected by the government. This amount, which is lost to both consumers and the government, is called the **Dead-weight loss.**

Factors of production: Land, labor, raw materials, machines, and buildings.

Flat grants: A system of intergovernmental aid to school districts whereby the central government sends each district a predetermined dollar amount per pupil enrolled or in attendance.

Foundation plan: A system of intergovernmental aid to school districts whereby the central government pays each district a proportion of some prespecified dollar amount per pupil. The proportion of that fixed amount paid to a district varies inversely with the district's tax base per pupil relative to the state average tax base per pupil.

General equilibrium model: A model representing the relationship between the prices of several goods and the demands and supplies of each of those goods.

Guaranteed tax base: A system of intergovernmental aid to school districts guaranteeing each district the equivalent of some prespecified (property) tax base per pupil. If the prespecified tax base per pupil is B^*, then a district with a tax base per pupil of $B \leq B^*$ and a tax rate of t would receive $\$t(B^* - B)$ in state aid.

Hedonic regression: A regression equation in which the dependent variable is the price of some good and the independent variables are the characteristics of that good.

Horizontal equity: The objective of the principle that households with equal abilities to pay should bear equal tax burdens.

Hypothesis: A tentative assertion made in order to draw out and test its logical or empirical consequences.

Impact aid: A federal intergovernmental grant program to aid school districts in proportion to the number of children of federal government employees the district serves.

Incidence of taxation: The distribution of the burden of a tax among economic actors, resulting in the reduction of that actor's (or group of actors') well-being or profits.

Independent variable: A variable whose value is determined by factors not included in a model.

Model: A set of assumptions (or postulates) constituting a simplified representation of (social or economic) relationships.

Municipal overburden hypothesis: The assertion that large cities, because they spend more per capita on nonschool public services than other types of jurisdictions, spend less on schools.

Normative economic theory: The branch of economics that develops criteria for evaluating the performance of an economy; also called **Welfare economics.**

Partial equilibrium model: A model representing the relationship between the price of a single good and the demand and supply of that good.

Percentage equalization: A system of intergovernmental aid to school districts under which the state pays a prespecified share of the expenditures of each school district. The percentage of any given district's total expenditures paid by the state is inversely proportional to the district's tax base per pupil relative to the state average tax base per pupil.

Power equalization: A system of intergovernmental aid to school districts guaranteeing that districts with equal tax rates will spend equal amounts per pupil.

Predictive economic theory: The branch of economics that generates qualitative predictions of the relationships among economic variables, usually in the form: if variable A increases, variable B tends to increase (or decrease) by an amount related to variables $C, D, E,$ and so on.

Present value: The amount that one would be willing to pay now in order to receive a stream of predetermined cash payments over some predetermined period.

Production technology: The totality of ways in which factors of production can be combined to produce some commodity.

Progressive tax: A tax that places a higher relative burden on high-income households than on low-income households.

Public good: A commodity such that one individual's consumption does not diminish the quantity available for others to consume.

Pupil weighting: An approach to state school aid formula design. Each type of student is assigned a certain weight. Districts are sent grants in aid in proportion to the total weight of students in the district.

Regression equation: A mathematical equation relating some dependent variable to a set of independent variables.

Regressive tax: A tax that places a higher relative burden on low-income households than on high-income households.

SMSA: Standard metropolitan statistical area.

Social welfare function: A mathematical statement representing some individual's social values.

Supply curve: A set of points, each representing the quantity of a good that would be brought to market for sale at a given price.

Tax price: The dollar amount a resident of a locality must pay in the form of increased taxes if total local public expenditures, expenditures per capita, or school expenditures per pupil are to increase by one dollar.

Utility: Subjective well-being or happiness.

Vertical equity: The objective of the principle that households with greater ability to pay should bear the greater tax burden.

Voucher: A document, issued to individuals, usually by a government, to be exchanged for a specific good.

Welfare economics: See **Normative economic theory.**

REFERENCES

Aaron, Henry J. 1975. *Who Pays the Property Tax? A New View.* Washington, D.C.: The Brookings Institution.

Abramowitz, S., and S. Rosenfeld. 1978. *Declining Enrollments: The Challenge of the Coming Decade.* Washington, D.C.: U.S. Government Printing Office.

Arrow, Kenneth J. 1971. "Equality in Public Expenditure." *Quarterly Journal of Economics* 85, no. 3 (August): 409–415.

Atkinson, A.B. 1970. "On the Measurement of Inequality." *Journal of Economic Theory* 2 (September): 244–263.

Atkinson, A. B., and J. E. Stiglitz. 1972. "The Structure of Indirect Taxation and Economic Efficiency." *Journal of Public Economics* 1, no. 1 (April): 97–119.

Barro, S.M. 1974. "The Impact of Intergovernmental Aid on Public School Spending." Unpublished doctoral dissertation, Stanford University.

Bergstrom, Theodore C., and Robert P. Goodman. 1973. "Private Demands for Public Goods." *The American Economic Review* 63, no. 3 (June): 280–296.

Berne, Robert, and Leanna Stiefel. 1979. "Taxpayer Equity in School Finance Reform." *Journal of Education Finance* 5 (Summer): 35–54.

Borcherding, Thomas E., and Robert T. Deacon. 1972. "The Demand for the Services of Non-Federal Governments." *The American Economic Review* 62, no. 5 (December): 891–901.

Brazer, Harvey E. 1974. "Adjusting for Differences Among School Districts in the Costs of Educational Inputs: A Feasibility Report." In *Selected Papers in School Finance: 1974,* edited by Esther O. Tron, pp. 89–133. Washington, D.C.: U.S. Office of Education.

Brown, Byron W., and Daniel H. Saks. 1975. "The Production and Distribution of Cognitive Skills within Schools." *Journal of Political Economy* 83, no. 3 (June): 571–593.

Brown, Byron W., and Daniel H. Saks. 1980. "Production Technologies and Resource Allocations within Classrooms and Schools." In *The Analysis of Educational Productivity, Vol. 1: Issues in Microanalysis,* edited by Robert Dreeben and J. Alan Thomas, pp. 53–117. Cambridge, Mass.: Ballinger Publishing Company.

Brueckner, Jan K. 1979. "Property Values, Local Public Expenditure and Economic Efficiency." *Journal of Public Economics* 11, no. 2 (April): 223–245.

Carroll, Stephen J. 1979. *The Search for Equity in School Finance: Results from Five States.* Santa Monica, Calif.: The Rand Corporation (R-2348-NIE).

Coons, John E., and Stephen D. Sugarman. 1978. *Education by Choice: The Case for Family Control.* Berkeley, Calif.: University of California Press.

Coons, J.E., W.H. Clune, and S.D. Sugarman. 1970. *Private Wealth and Public Education.* Cambridge, Mass.: Belknap Press.

Diamond, Peter A., and James A. Mirrlees. 1971. "Optimal Taxation and Public Production." *The American Economic Review* 61, no. 1 (March): 8–27.

Edel, Matthew, and Elliott Sclar. 1974. "Taxes, Spending, and Property Values: Supply Adjustment in a Tiebout-Oates Model." *Journal of Political Economy* 82, no. 5 (September/October): 941–954.

Education Commission of the States. 1975. *School Finance Reform: The Wherewithals.* Denver, Colo.

Ellickson, Bryan, Barry Fishman, and Peter A. Morrison. 1977. *Economic Analysis of Urban Housing Markets: A New Approach.* Santa Monica, Calif.: The Rand Corporation (R-2024-NSF).

Feldstein, Martin S. 1975. "Wealth Neutrality and Local Choice in Public Education," *The American Economic Review* 65, no. 1 (March): 75–89.

Friedman, Milton. 1962. *Capitalism and Freedom.* Chicago: University of Chicago Press.

Gittell, Marilyn, T. Edward Hollander, and William S. Vincent. 1970. "Fiscal Status and School Policy Making in Six Large School Districts." In *The Politics of Education at the Local, State and Federal Levels,* edited by Michael W. Kirst, pp. 33–73. Berkeley, Calif.: McCutchan Publishing Corporation.

Gurwitz, Aaron S. 1980. "The Capitalization of School Finance Reform." *Journal of Educational Finance* 5, no. 3 (Winter): 297–319.

Hamilton, Alexander, James Madison, and John Jay. 1961. *The Federalist Papers.* New York: The New American Library.

Hamilton, Bruce W. 1976. "Capitalization of Intrajurisdictional Differences in Local Tax Prices." *The American Economic Review* 66, no. 5 (December): 743–753.

Harberger, Arnold C. 1962. "The Incidence of the Corporation Income Tax." *Journal of Political Economy* 70 (June): 215–240.

Harberger, Arnold C. 1971. "Three Basic Postulates for Applied Welfare Economics: An Interpretative Essay." *Journal of Economic Literature* 9, no. 3 (September): 785–797.

Inman, Robert P. 1978. "Optimal Fiscal Reform of Metropolitan Schools: Some Simulation Results." *The American Economic Review* 68, no. 1 (March): 107–122.

Ladd, Helen F. 1975. "Local Education Expenditures, Fiscal Capacity, and the Composition of the Property Tax Base." *National Tax Journal* 28, no. 2 (June): 145–158.

MacKinnon, J. 1974. "Urban General Equilibrium Models and Simplicial Search." *Journal of Urban Economics* 1, no. 2 (April): 161–183.

McClure, C.E. 1975. "General Equilibrium Incidence Analysis." *Journal of Public Economics* 4, no. 2 (February): 125–161.

Netzer, Dick. 1974. "State Education Aid and School Tax Efforts in Large Cities." In *Selected Papers in School Finance: 1974,* edited by Esther O. Tron, pp. 135–232. Washington, D.C.: U.S. Office of Education.

Newachek, Paul W. 1979. "Capitalization: The Price of School Finance Reform." *Policy Analysis* 5, no. 1 (Winter): 21–36.

Oates, Wallace E. 1969. "The Effects of Property Taxes and Local Spending on Property Values: An Empirical Study of Tax Capitalization and the Tiebout Hypothesis." *Journal of Political Economy* 77 (November/December): 957–971.

Ordeshook, Peter C., ed. 1978. *Game Theory and Political Science.* New York: New York University Press.

Park, Rolla Edward, and Stephen J. Carroll. 1979. *The Search for Equity in School Finance: Michigan School District Response to a Guaranteed Tax Base.* Santa Monica, Calif.: The Rand Corporation (R-2392-NIE/HEW).

Pascal, Anthony H., et al. 1979. *Fiscal Containment of Local and State Government.* Santa Monica, Calif.: The Rand Corporation (R-2494-FF/RC).

Perkins, George M. 1977. "The Demand for Local Public Goods: Elasticities of Demand for Own Price, Cross Prices, and Income." *National Tax Journal* 30, no. 4 (December): 411–422.

Salisbury, Robert H. 1970. "Schools and Politics in the Big City." In *The Politics of Education at the Local, State and Federal Levels,* edited by Michael W. Kirst, pp. 17–32. Berkeley, Calif.: McCutchan Publishing Corporation.

Shoven, John B., and John Whalley. 1972. "A General Equilibrium Calculation of the Effects of Differential Taxation of Income from Capital in the U.S." *Journal of Public Economics* 1, no. 3/4 (November): 281–321.

Smith, Adam. 1937. *The Wealth of Nations.* Modern Library Edition. New York: Random House.

Supreme Court of the State of New York. 1974. "Post-Trial Review of the Evidence for Plaintiffs-Intervenors." *Levittown v. Nyquist* (Index No. 8208/74).

Supreme Court of the United States. *Brown v. Board of Education.* 347 U.S. 483, 1954.

Summers, Anita A., and Barbara L. Wolfe. 1977. "Do Schools Make a Difference?" *The American Economic Review* 67, no. 4 (September): 639–652.

Tiebout, Charles M. 1956. "A Pure Theory of Local Expenditures." *Journal of Political Economy* 65 (October): 416–424.

Wendling, Wayne. 1979. *Expenditures and Tax Capitalization: Its Relation to School Finance and Tax Reform.* Denver, Colo.: Education Commission of the States.

Wise, Arthur E. 1979. *Legislated Learning.* Berkeley, Calif.: University of California Press.

RAND EDUCATIONAL POLICY STUDIES

PUBLISHED

Averch, Harvey A., et al. 1974. *How Effective is Schooling? A Critical Review of Research*. Englewood Cliffs, N.J.: Educational Technology Publications.

Carpenter-Huffman, P., et al. 1974. *Change in Education: Insights from Performance Contracting*. Cambridge, Mass.: Ballinger Publishing Company.

Crain, Robert L., et al. 1981. *Making Desegregation Work: How Schools Create Social Climates*. Cambridge, Mass.: Ballinger Publishing Company.

Elmore, Richard, and Milbrey W. McLaughlin. 1982. *Reform and Retrenchment: The Politics of California School Finance Reform*. Cambridge, Mass.: Ballinger Publishing Company.

Gurwitz, Aaron S. 1982. *The Economics of Public School Finance*. Cambridge, Mass.: Ballinger Publishing Company.

McLaughlin, Milbrey W. 1975. *Evaluation and Reform: The Elementary and Secondary Education Act of 1965. Title I*. Cambridge, Mass.: Ballinger Publishing Company.

Pincus, John (ed.). 1974. *School Finance in Transition: The Courts and Educational Reform*. Cambridge, Mass.: Ballinger Publishing Company.

Timpane, Michael (ed.). 1978. *The Federal Interest in Financing Schooling*. Cambridge, Mass.: Ballinger Publishing Company.

OTHER RAND BOOKS IN EDUCATION

Bruno, James E., (Ed.) *Emerging Issues in Education: Policy Implications for the Schools.* Lexington, Mass.: D.C. Heath and Company, 1972.

Coleman, James S. and Nancy L. Karweit. *Information Systems and Performance Measures in Schools.* Englewood Cliffs, New Jersey: Educational Technology Publications, 1972.

Haggart, Sue A. (Ed.) *Program Budgeting for School District Planning.* Englewood Cliffs, New Jersey: Educational Technology Publications, 1972.

Levien, Roger E. *The Emerging Technology: Instructional Uses of The Computer in Higher Education.* New York: McGraw-Hill Book Company, 1972.

INDEX